I0790428

The Light After Loss

SANDY BODEAU

The Light After Loss

How the power of social media is breaking the silence around miscarriage

To my sweet Richard for choosing me every day as we walked through darkness and for giving me the brightest light that ever was: our beautiful children, Lennox Ryan and Mara Victoria.

TABLE OF CONTENTS

FOREWORD

Luz María Doria

I have never written about this. I had never even explained it as I want to explain it here. And I have to confess that it may be way more difficult than I anticipated. Sandy's invitation to write this foreword came to me a couple of months ago and I never found the perfect time to start writing it.

But I know why. I will start sharing my story here and tell you all about the process that I went through when I lost my baby. This is for those of you who have suffered a loss. I do not want you to feel alone. I do not want you to feel that your life is over. I want you to understand that unborn babies never die. They will always live in the heart of their mothers. The hearts of those moms they never got to meet, but that I am sure they chose themselves to leave a big mark in their hearts.

Tomás was going to be Dominique's little brother. The pregnancy came at a very special moment in our lives because, unlike Dominique - who was a miracle after almost 7 years of trying to have a baby - Tomas was the result of tests that proved that my hormones were not working as they should and that was why I was not able to get pregnant. The damned fear, before having Dominique, prevented me from going to the doctor to get tested to see what was wrong. But once my little girl was born, I told my doctor about my fears and she agreed to run some tests.

I took care of myself like never before. This pregnancy was supervised. Everything had to go very well. My fridge was full of healthy foods. I started drinking orange juice with carrots and eating fruits. I was so excited that my daughter was going to have a little brother.

I made all the plans in the world. I promised myself that I was going to disconnect completely during my maternity leave, since I never did that 100% during Dominique's. It would be a moment just for me and my baby.

Everything had to go well. The doctor agreed. The results of my exams were perfect. Everything was going so well that there was, according to her, no reason to continue with the hormones. I believed her.

And, suddenly, one day in spite of already being 14 weeks along, I stopped feeling pregnant. "All pregnancies are not the same," people repeated. In the routine exam, it was reconfirmed. "Everything is fine. All pregnancies are not the same."

That same day in the doctor's office I asked for an ultrasound and they told me that I was not due for one. I demanded it. I said I would pay for it if the insurance didn't cover it. They finally agreed. While the technician was looking at the screen, I asked her if everything was OK with my baby. "I can't tell you anything," she replied with a somber look. "The doctor will talk to you in a minute."

The doctor entered the room and simply asked: "How did you know that something was wrong?" She asked me with such coldness that broke my heart into little pieces. My baby's heartbeat had stopped. My suspicions were true. I was no longer pregnant. The doctor kept talking as my heart kept breaking for the loss of our little Tomás. "Yes, the embryo stopped growing," she proceeded to explain. "We have to clean all the remains of the pregnancy. But you have to wait until Monday because there is no space at the hospital until then."

I left the doctor's office and called my husband. I explained everything to him as I cried uncontrollably. I then called Sonia, my assistant, so she could let everyone know. If there is something worse than losing a baby, it is having people ask how the pregnancy is going once the pregnancy is gone. I also didn't want anyone to give me their condolences.

My dad called me and explained the statistics and tried to convince me that it was better that it had happened now than learning about a complication later on. But I was full of pain and anger. Very angry.

It hurt to tell Dominique that her little brother was not going to come. It made me angry to have to wait for days with that little bit of life inside my body. A friend of mine who is a gynecologist called me to tell me that he did not understand why my doctor had stopped my hormone treatment, since this was a way of feeding my baby.

On Monday, I got up and went to church. I gave God my pain and 4 hours later I woke up in the hospital after a general anesthetic. I felt completely empty. "That shouldn't have happened to you," a friend told me recklessly. "After all you have gone through to get pregnant". Maybe her way of victimizing me made me react. It was then that I understood that I had to keep going for my daughter. I also had to keep going for my husband – whose pain I had selfishly ignored. But I also understood that that inexplicable pain that accentuated when I opened the fridge and remembered that I should no longer take care of myself for that little face I never knew would always live in me.

It's been almost 20 years. And even though we have never spoken about this again in our house, I always tell all my young friends that they need to face their fears, check their hormones and seek help when trying to get pregnant. And every Sunday, at Mass, I pray for my little son who was never born.

Luz María Doria
Author of "La Mujer de Mis Sueños" and "Tu Momento Estelar"
and executive producer at Despierta América

CHAPTER 1

THE POWER OF A VERY SIMPLE QUESTION

August 25, 2018

I took a deep breath before stepping into the elevator that would take me to the Facebook offices in Miami. This was not where I wanted to be. It had been 10 days since my post that told the world I had lost another baby. It was my fourth loss.

Where I wanted to be was back at home in the safety of my room, hiding in bed with the covers pulled up around me; crying as my mom took care of my son. But my husband had convinced me that this would be good for me, since I would be surrounded by people that cared about me. Still, I was truly dreading walking into that conference room.

This was the kind of meeting where I would know almost everyone. The room would be full of my friends and colleagues. Basically, it would be many of the very same people that I wanted to hide from right now. The RSVP had been sent in before my miscarriage, but that seemed long ago. Up until the moment that I'd actually gotten in my car to go, I hadn't been able to imagine seeing anyone who knew what had happened to me. And now I was terrified that I would be spending the whole morning with an entire room full of them.

But here I was, the first person in the conference room along with our host, Ignacio. Ignacio de los Reyes was a warm and charming fellow Spaniard. It was a relief to learn that we had something in common. And it was a gift that he knew nothing about the ordeal that I had recently been through. His warm welcome made me forget about my nerves a little bit as we chatted about how long we both had been in the U.S. He told me all about why he loved San Francisco, the city he now called home. It was a welcome change from the recurring thoughts that had been circling my head for the past two weeks.

As we talked, people that I knew kept walking into the room. Each time someone entered, I physically hid behind Ignacio, using the conversation as a way to not be noticed. This was no easy task, since I stand well over 6'1" when I wear high heels. But I was determined, and apparently successful.

Now it was time to go find a place to sit and watch the presentation. With my heart beating out of my chest, I walked towards the chairs. This is one of the hardest feelings to deal with after a miscarriage. Thinking that all eyes are on you. It felt as if my "Hi, my name is…" label actually read: "Hi, my body is failing me."

As soon as we sat down, my friend Jeannette Kaplun began walking towards me. My heart started to beat even faster. "Please, do not cry," I told myself over and over. Jeannette opened her arms and wrapped them around me warmly as she whispered in my ear: "How are you doing?" My heart started to slow down. No tears sprung up. I felt relieved and at peace. "I am going to be okay," I told her. She gave me a big smile and replied: "I know you will."

To this day, Jeannette surely does not realize the impact of her actions at that moment. I was able to breathe calmly through the meeting. And I was able to look the rest of my friends in the eye without fear of breaking down. To my welcome surprise, I was even able to enjoy the meeting!

It had never been easy for me to identify what I wanted or needed from others after my losses. All I had really learned from my previous experiences was that people do not know how to act when they see you for the first time after a miscarriage. Most often they say nothing. It is a subject not spoken about and the silence is deafening. And the awkwardness of that always made me feel invisible.

Jeannette was the first person to teach me what was needed in that situation. What was needed was a normal reaction. It was a friend who would simply ask: "How are you doing?" It was for people to acknowledge that I was going through a very hard time. What I did not need were the silences or awkward encounters. I needed normalcy. Loss is a part of life and miscarriage is no different. I simply needed to be treated like any other person would be treated while going through a terribly painful loss.

This encounter with my friend Jeannette, and the experience that day at Facebook, was pivotal. It marked a before and after in my approach towards sharing my story and my journey to successfully carry another pregnancy after having my beautiful son. While I had previously been open about my miscarriages, it was on that day that it became clear to me that I wanted to have a bigger voice. It was no longer only about sharing my journey to let others know that they were not alone. Jeannette's actions made me realize that I needed to speak to a broader audience.

Women who faced the pain of losing a baby after miscarriage were suffering in silence. They felt isolated and alone. I needed to share my story and share the lessons I was learning. That way, the friends and loved ones of women facing fertility issues would begin to see how they could help them heal during that very painful journey.

As I write this, I am eight months pregnant with my daughter. If you are still going through your infertility season, it would be normal to think that it is because I am pregnant that I can talk about finding light after loss. While the pregnancy with my daughter is the happy ending to one of the toughest battles of my life, I found the light well before I got pregnant with her.

My light came because of women like you and me. It was women who had suffered miscarriages or were struggling to get pregnant that helped me find the light in my darkest hours. Comment after comment and private message after private message on my Instagram account, those women showed me the light. And it was a light so bright that it propelled me forward when I felt absolutely powerless and lost. It was a light that gave me a voice that the world was listening to.

Those women gave me a purpose to be able to make sense of my painful journey. They are the driving force behind this book. It is not a book about me. It is a book about a topic that continues to be a huge taboo in our society.

Each chapter begins with a post from my Instagram account and a select comment from a follower. And each one ends with a story from among the many that my Instagram followers shared with me. It is my hope that every single one of these chapters helps you begin to find your own light. Or to help someone else find theirs.

Believe me, the light does not only appear when you succeed. There is, indeed, a lot of beauty in finding the light within the pain.

NOELIA'S STORY

I was 28 years old when I got pregnant for the first time. I was so excited. Then, one morning at 12 weeks gestation, I saw a little bit of blood on the toilet paper while using the bathroom. It was just a little, but it scared me enough to go to the hospital. A vaginal ultrasound confirmed that I had a blighted ovum. I did not even know what that meant! The doctor explained to me that the placenta had been created but there was nothing else inside my uterus.

After the initial shock, it only got more difficult. I had to go to the hospital the next day to be prescribed a pill that would help me eliminate the remaining tissue from the unsuccessful pregnancy. On that day, we received more shocking news. My uterus was actually not empty. They, indeed, found a 12-week-old fetus without a heartbeat.

I went home even more devastated than I had left. I had to take three pills, and just 20 minutes after taking the first one, I started having completely unexpected contractions. The contraction pain felt like someone was stabbing me in the back and left me, literally, lying on the floor from it. Two hours later, I was unable to move from the toilet due to pain as I bled non-stop. I literally felt as if my guts were being emptied. Then I heard a big "thump" in the water, and I knew exactly what it was. Shocked, I just flushed the toilet, unable to look.

Three months later, I was pregnant again. And, again, at six weeks of pregnancy, I started bleeding. I again headed to the hospital, where they quickly determined that it was too early for a heartbeat and I was sent home. I decided to take a voluntary leave from work, so I could focus on resting. At 10 weeks, it was confirmed during a regular visit that my baby had stopped growing at eight weeks. Naked on the bottom half of my body, I had to jump from the bed to console my husband who literally collapsed on his knees crying after hearing the news.

And again, more pills. This time, I was just walking around the house when I felt the fetus coming out from me and into my panties. I screamed and cried for my mom's help as I walked to the bathroom. I begged her to take the panties from me as I covered my face.

I constantly wondered "why me?" to which my mom replied, "Keep praying, everything will be okay." Deep inside of me I just felt that God had abandoned me.

Join the movement. Share these stories so that we all have a voice. #TheLightAfterLoss

- @siramara
- Sandy Bodeau
- @sanbodeau

CHAPTER 2

BREAKING THROUGH DARKNESS

December 29, 2015

'When a new day begins, dare to smile gratefully.
When there is darkness, dare to be the first to shine a light.
When there is injustice, dare to be the first to condemn it.
When something seems difficult, dare to do it anyway.

When life seems to beat you down, dare to fight back.
When there seems to be no hope, dare to find some.
When you're feeling tired, dare to keep going
When times are tough, dare to be tougher.

When love hurts you, dare to love again.
When someone is hurting, dare to help them heal.
When another is lost, dare to help them find the way.
When a friend falls, dare to be the first to extend a hand.

When you cross paths with another, dare to make them smile.
When you feel great, dare to help someone else feel great too.
When the day has ended, dare to feel as you've done your best.
Dare to be the best you can.'

Steve Maraboli, Life, the Truth, and Being Free

"Such a wonderful message. But, of course, it is" @*beautifulmiami*

I had gone into hiding on social media and people were starting to notice. At the time, posting every day was my norm. My seven day break started to raise questions, particularly among my most loyal followers. The holidays helped to explain a bit, but disappearing like that was not like me. The truth was it was not holiday celebrations that kept me away. It was sadness, and pain, and bleeding that did not stop for well over a week and required a second hospital visit.

It was my first pregnancy. There had been some spotting, and even some bleeding at the start of the pregnancy. But what happened the day of the miscarriage is still hard to comprehend. It was one of the few times in my life that I felt mortally vulnerable.

My Instagram community knows that I had been diagnosed with sickle cell anemia as a young girl. Due to this diagnosis, I had chosen a very healthy lifestyle throughout my life. That led me to become a strong and healthy athlete. But there in the hospital, my awareness shifted from my healthy body to a vulnerable one that was barely recognizable.

I lost a lot of blood that day – more than anyone realized at the time. Some before reaching the hospital, some in the ER, some as we awaited the ultrasound, and still more as we awaited the results. Individually, any member of the medical team probably thought it was a lot. But only my husband and I knew it had been happening at every stop during the entire day. And at the time, in the moment, we did not have a perspective to understand how bad it was.

What I knew, simply, was that I was scared. I feared I had lost my baby. My body certainly knew there was a problem, and the messages it was sending made me fearful that something had gone terribly wrong.

By the time the doctor confirmed that my baby was gone and that a D&C would be required, I was not comfortable letting them give me anesthesia. My body was increasingly telling me that something was not right. Something in my heart told me that if I were to go under, there was a chance I would not come out of it.

It would be nice if I could say that the D&C without anesthesia was not too bad. But that is simply not true. I got through it with my husband holding my hand and speaking calmly to me. The look in his eyes told me I was doing well. I still remember it vividly, in many ways. But parts of it are simply a blur of pain, colors, and images of everything going on around me. Never in my life had I experienced pain like that. It was a pain so intense that it made me forget, for those very long minutes, that my heart was broken from the loss of what was supposed to be our first baby.

Having the D&C without anesthesia was the right decision, and I have no regrets. I was not confident that I could go into surgery and wake up afterward. But I knew I was strong enough to endure the pain and walk out of the hospital after the procedure. And the alternative was not a risk I was willing to take.

In total, about eight hours had gone by from the moment we arrived at the hospital to the moment my husband pushed me out in a wheelchair to go home. We went through the same hallways, and I saw the same faces that had greeted me when I'd arrived. Life had continued, with no awareness of the changes that had happened while we were inside. It was a strikingly surreal experience.

As life had carried on unaware that day, I had lost a child. But I had also gained perspective. And a great deal of respect from my husband for the strength he saw in me.

PAULA'S STORY

Hi! I wanted to share this with you. I had a miscarriage. We heard a heartbeat at six weeks and three days. Five days later, I started having back pain and cramps. I went to the doctor and an ultrasound confirmed that the heart had stopped beating. I had a D&C yesterday.

I am devastated but, in the midst of it all, I have managed to keep my hopes up and thank God. But this time around and after two previous miscarriages, this has killed us. My husband and I have cried so much in the last few days. It does not seem real. This is my third recurrent miscarriage. Even though I already have two children, it is still painful.

I think that we are ready to see a specialist. My husband got tested and his sperm is perfect. So, it must be me or some kind of event that just happens. But I need answers. We want to keep trying. I have faith that we will have another baby.

You sharing your experience has given me so much hope. I saw your post when you announced your pregnancy, and I was genuinely happy for you, and I said: "God if you did it for her, you will do that miracle for me, too." I wanted you to know that your post gave me hope and it will continue to do so. God wanted me to see that post that day.

———

Join the movement. Share these stories so that we all have a voice. #TheLightAfterLoss

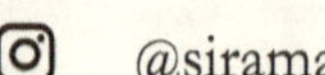

@siramara

Sandy Bodeau

@sanbodeau

CHAPTER 3

ALWAYS THANKFUL

December 31, 2015

Dear 2015,

Thank you for being the year that brought me my very own fashion segment on national TV. Every new year comes with blessings I could have never imagined, so I am READY for you, 2016.

"Can't wait to see what's next for you, San. You are a true star."

Just 10 days after my first miscarriage, I was 'back in business.' From the outside, everything seemed to be normal. There I was, back in warrior mode, without a hint that anything bad had happened. But in this message there was a thankfulness that only my husband and I understood at the time.

In spite of the pain I was going through, I was indeed ending the year with a grateful heart. Being grateful is something that I always try to focus on. And this situation was no different. Losing a child is never easy. In fact, it is devastating. But the unique circumstances made it easier to process compared to the losses that followed. And not because it was my first.

When we got home from the hospital that night, I began to process what had happened. My mind kept replaying the many times that a nurse had replace the blood-soaked sheets as we waited for tests and results. That was one of the scariest experiences of my life. More than once I was overcome by the feeling that I would die that day. So, sitting at home that night with my husband by my side, I was truly grateful that I was safe. I was alive. I had survived.

Of course we felt the loss. We had already begun to see ourselves as parents. This was an unplanned pregnancy, but we embraced it and were excited about it from the get-go. We marveled at the miracle of life the first (and last) time we saw our baby's heartbeat in an ultrasound. A little heart created by our love was beating inside my body. Our family was growing and we were on an amazing journey together. Our future was unfolding before our eyes. Until it wasn't.

There is something about facing your own mortality that makes you realize that you do not always control your future. That we sometimes need to be thankful for what did not happen, rather than the loss that did happen. It was from that perspective that I started to look at my miscarriage from that day forward.

That does not mean that I was not also tremendously shaken. Never will I forget the moment I fainted from having lost so much blood. My body was shutting down. It could not take any more of the trauma that had been going on non-stop for several hours.

Right before losing consciousness, I grabbed the nurse's hand – I still remember her name was Rose – and asked her, "Am I going to die?" It was not that I was being dramatic or paranoid. This simply felt like it was the end for me. She looked me in the eyes and said: "No, honey. Of course not. Nobody is dying here today."

Months and months later, those words still echoed in my mind each time I thought about that day. Rose had promised me that nobody was going to die that day, but she was wrong. My first baby died that day, in fact he or she was already dead as Rose was making that promise. It was only with time that I fully understood what her words meant.

In general, the world does not think of miscarriage as a death. Rose was sweet. She was kind. She was a great professional that day and I am forever thankful for her. But she missed a very important point. Someone did die that day.

Not only that, something inside of me also died after that first miscarriage. In its place was an indescribable void. It happens within hours. Your mind goes through the shock of processing that one minute you were pregnant and the next you were not. It is a striking contrast between the instantaneous joy you feel when you learn you are pregnant and the profound sadness you feel when you experience miscarriage. It is one of the most brutal feelings to process.

So here I found myself on the eve of the new year. The past few weeks had been a whirlwind. Each day I laid in bed, crying and bleeding. There was a gaping hole cut into my heart that barely allowed me to breathe. And yet, while this miscarriage was a devastating loss, the perspective of having walked out of that hospital alive helped to soften the blow.

So on this New Year's Eve, I was genuinely grateful. Grateful for my life, for my love, and for my career. And I was grateful for the potential future that was before me. I faced the new year with a grateful heart, even as I grappled with a deep sorrow. The pain had not disappeared. It had just settled in and become part of my being. I accepted it for what it was. Something you learn to live with, but that never, ever leaves you.

ELISABETH'S STORY

Recently, I was faced with the saddest of truths. I learned that I had lost my baby at two months of pregnancy. I was so sad. To be honest, your story was the first that came to mind. I thought of your openness in sharing your experiences, and that helped ease my thoughts. Thinking of how you have struggled so much and have still kept the faith. And now you have your girl on the way. I truly want to thank you for always being so open and real and wish nothing but happiness and joy for you and your family.

———

Join the movement. Share these stories so that we all have a voice. #TheLightAfterLoss

⬛ @siramara
⬛ Sandy Bodeau
⬛ @sanbodeau

CHAPTER 4

I GOT IT FROM MY MAMA

May 8, 2016

'I got it from my Mama'

Absolutely everything I am. Happy Mother's Day, my darlings! #MothersDay

"Enjoy your Mother's Day, my girl."

That was my post on my Instagram account on my first Mother's Day post-miscarriage. The day that was supposed to have been my first Mother's Day. Well, my first mama-to-be day. Instead, it was Bloody Marys and brunch with my favorite chef, my husband. We made the best of the day and spent it in quiet isolation, curled up on the couch and reminiscing about those eventful days just a few months earlier.

The months that had gone by helped me to look at those traumatic moments from a calm place. The pain was still there, but I was able to look at what had happened as a terrible isolated event. So much so, we were already trying to have another baby. The trauma from the first miscarriage was much more physical than emotional. Emotionally, I was ready to try to get pregnant again. And I was actually convinced that it would happen soon.

The doctor had advised me to wait two full cycles after getting my period back before trying to get pregnant again. My period came back in

January, and we started trying to get pregnant again in March. Two cycles. My heart, my head and my body were ready. I had no fears.

It was two weeks after that Mother's Day post that I got pregnant with my son, Lennox. Getting pregnant so quickly never felt like luck. It was my ability to feel at peace after that first pregnancy that I attributed to the quick success. My continued calm I attributed to that same peace, and the reassurance of my doctor. She assured me that there was no reason to fear a second miscarriage, explaining that first pregnancies have a very high chance of miscarriage. Armed with my doctor's affirmation, I was ready to put that episode behind me and embrace my new pregnancy.

But it was a rough pregnancy. I suffered from tremendous nausea for most of the first four months of the pregnancy. Right after the nausea subsided, I started having paralyzing sciatica pain. That was followed by the discovery that I had an additional blood disorder, alpha thalassemia. When I truly thought that I could not face any more physical challenges, I was diagnosed with gestational diabetes. That was a huge blow, and a shock to both me and my doctor, because I take great pride in my healthy lifestyle. The icing on the cake was the excruciating rib pain I endured courtesy of the kicks from my almost 10-pound baby.

But although my pregnancy with Lennox was physically challenging, I embraced every second of it. I marveled at the miracle of life each time I saw an ultrasound or felt him moving in my belly. It was incredible to realize a tiny human was growing inside of me. I fell in love with the entire process. And the thought of miscarriage did not cross my mind once.

Nine months after that post on Mother's Day, Lennox was born. Seeing what a challenge pregnancy had been for my body, I had sworn that I would only have one child. But I changed my mind almost as soon as Lennox came along. My brother came from Spain to help us adapt to our new life. It was then that I remembered the importance of siblings as a support system. Suddenly, I felt the need to give my sweet boy a sibling close in age that could provide that support system that had been so essential to me throughout my life.

At my 6-weeks postpartum appointment, with my c-section scar still healing, I asked the doctor when we could start trying to have another baby. "At least six months". Okay. It was decided. We would start trying as soon as we could. Convinced that it would not happen for a while, we stopped taking precautions when Lennox was five-months-old. To our absolute shock, I got pregnant on the first try! We were ELATED! We were having another baby. Our family would be complete in nine months and Lennox would get to grow up with a best friend!

RUTH'S STORY

I met my ex-husband in 2013, a little over a year after arriving in the U.S. Everything was incredible. We got married in 2014. I was 34-years-old. Family and friends quickly started asking "When will you guys have children?" What nobody knew was that, just a few months after getting married, there was a lot of hidden stress and illness. I was suffering from hyperthyroidism and psoriasis, which caused lots of rejection from my husband. In addition to his rejection to my physical changes, he also resented me for being unable to get pregnant due to the issues that thyroid problems cause hormonally.

The day came when I found the courage to separate, and I felt like I had gotten rid of a great burden in my life. My psoriasis started to get better and doctors lowered the dose of my thyroid medication every month. I still thought that I would never be able to get pregnant.

Then, I met my current partner. We have a long distance relationship. A few months after we began dating, he came to spend some time with me and I got pregnant. I could not believe it! I was so shocked. I did not tell anybody. I was so excited but also too guarded to share. I did not even share it with my boyfriend. When I finally began to feel ready to tell him, it was too late. After a few days of cramping and bleeding, I lost my baby at six weeks of pregnancy. I have not been able to get pregnant again, but I still have hope that I will one day be blessed to become a mother and create a family with my boyfriend.

Join the movement. Share these stories so
that we all have a voice. #TheLightAfterLoss
🄾   @siramara
🄵   Sandy Bodeau
🄱   @sanbodeau

CHAPTER 5

GONE BUT NOT FORGOTTEN

August 13, 2017

[POST REMOVED]

Having faced the loss of my father as a young girl and, shortly thereafter, my beloved Abuela (my maternal grandmother), I know a few things about loss. I lost my father overnight. He was alive one day and gone the next. At the time, I believed that there could not be a worse way to lose a loved one.

Just three years later, I lost my Abuela. This loss was very different. She was sick for about three months prior to her passing. While there are many aspects of shock in losing a loved one as suddenly as I lost my father, it is also heart-wrenching to watch the life slowly fade from the body of someone as important as my Abuela was to me. It became clear to me then that a loss is something you can never really prepare for.

What I also learned through those losses is that it does not really ever get better. You continue to grieve and miss them terribly. You just get better at dealing with the pain of the loss. Part of the healing is accepting that the pain is not going to go away. Part of that is choosing to take steps forward and embracing what you do have instead of constantly thinking about what you lost.

Just a week before posting the now removed Instagram post, I had begun to convince my husband to let me announce that we were expecting a baby. He was very hesitant. He said that he was superstitious, but I think he was just trying to protect my heart, and his own.

To reassure him, I showed him the statistics. The chances of miscarriage at nine weeks of pregnancy after hearing a heartbeat were just 4%. For me, it could have been 20% and it would not have mattered. I was convinced that my first miscarriage had been an isolated event. Lennox's birth had proven that. Miscarriage would never happen to us again. But I wanted my husband not to stress about announcing too early. The odds were overwhelmingly in our favor. We were not part of that 4%.

Hesitantly, my husband agreed to announce. My post that day was a picture of Lennox wearing a shirt that said 'Promoted to Big Brother.' Dozens and dozens of messages poured in. People were incredibly happy for us, and I was thrilled to get to share another pregnancy journey with my social media community.

The bleeding started exactly 24 hours after that announcement. I spent some time going through Google trying to find reasons for my bleeding that would tell me that it had nothing to do with a miscarriage. But the bleeding got worse, so we decided to go to the doctor.

At the doctor's office, they saw the baby and a heartbeat. The doctor also found blood in my gestational sac. He advised me to go home and rest until I was no longer bleeding. "You are threatening," he said. It was unsettling, but I was still certain that this was just another one of those stories people share about scares in the early stages of pregnancy.

A couple of hours after getting home, the bleeding intensified. Then came the cramping and the passing of blood clots. Each time I went to the bathroom and looked down to see a bloody piece of toilet paper, I cried uncontrollably. It was happening again. I was miscarrying.

The next few hours were spent passing tissue non-stop. Crying in my mama's arms. Sobbing on the bathroom floor while my husband held me. How was this happening again? I had just had a child! I knew my body could carry a healthy pregnancy! Was my son's pregnancy a fluke? Was my body, indeed, a broken machine? After a horrible night of blood and tears, it was confirmed in the morning that we had lost the baby.

The beautiful picture of Lennox in his 'Promoted to Big Brother' shirt was taken down from Instagram, along with my announcement and the wonderful comments from friends, family, and followers. But taking down the story would not undo what had been done. The genie was out of the bottle and it was not going back in.

PENELOPE'S STORY

I have been pregnant twice and I have lost both babies. My first loss was at five months and the second one at seven months. My heart is broken. I want to be a mother, but I am not sure that I have the strength to overcome the fear of another loss. Then, I think about how you kept the faith loss after loss, and I think that I may be able to try again one day. For now, I want to thank you for sharing your story. If I ever find the strength to try again, it will be in great part thanks to having found your Instagram posts. Your vulnerability is going to help so many women. It already is doing so. Thank you!

Join the movement. Share these stories so that we all have a voice. #TheLightAfterLoss
- @siramara
- Sandy Bodeau
- @sanbodeau

CHAPTER 6

THERE IS NO EASY WAY TO SAY IT

August 17, 2017

Is it easier to say it two days later or two months later? There's no 'easy' now and there won't be 'easy' later in sharing that your pregnancy ended abruptly & shockingly. You choose to take a deep breath and you say it. You choose to embrace the light of a new day. You choose to continue to live the beautiful life you've built. You choose to look at your marvelous son and smile because he's the happiest little human and sadness is just not an option around him. You choose to hold onto the words 'it was not a healthy pregnancy' to logically find peace within the sadness. You choose good instead of bad because you have always known that the simple fact of having that option makes you extremely fortunate. #YouChoose

{I'll 'see' you soon, my beloved virtual family}

"I'm so sorry dear ... truly. From one woman to another ...especially given the reasons I've already shared with you ...my thoughts and prayers are with you."

The post announcing my pregnancy had been removed, but there were still congratulations pouring in. There were also well-intentioned messages of concern from those who had noticed the removal of the announcement post and my cryptic post about surviving the storm that I had done the day before.

My husband had already reached out to some of my closest friends to tell them. The ones I knew could not be made to wait and worry about me. They were also the ones I could not bear to hear the kind words and affirmations from. It was hard to imagine how, at any point, I could even begin to find the words to tell them that my baby was gone. So that was a task I left to my husband. He gladly continued to reach out to everyone so I could focus on allowing myself to grieve in peace.

As much as it was great to have my husband handling the private sharing of our loss, this time it was a bigger audience that was worried. Over the years, I had developed some strong bonds with Instagram friends and followers. Our very public announcement just a few days prior could be removed, but never taken back. This was not a private loss, this was a public failure. At least that is how it felt. Within days, I went from presenting myself victorious to having to admit that I had failed myself and my family.

There was the pain, and then there was the guilt. My husband had agreed to announce even though he did not feel ready to share. It was me who had pushed him and that ate me from the inside. Not only had I put myself in a horrible position by announcing too early, but I had also put him in that position. Not only did I worry about how the public reaction would affect me, I had brought him into that. I deserved it but he did not.

It is probably obvious to you, reading this, that this was not how my husband felt. He was simply worried about me. And probably more than a little baffled at the number of times I sobbed and said, "I am sorry." But there is something so personal about losing a baby, that you cannot help but find ways to blame yourself.

Even as I drowned in my tears and my sadness, I knew that I had to choose, once again, how to deal with a loss. What advice would I give to a friend if they reached out for guidance? That advice would be to understand that the pain will not suddenly disappear. To remember all that is beautiful in life. And above all, to allow themselves ample time to grieve. Grieving is important. So that was my private plan.

Publicly, I was forced to talk about what had happened. That was clearly unavoidable. The very public announcement about the successful pregnancy now seemed to require an update of the unfortunate turn of events that had followed. It was me who had told everyone about my pregnancy. Now, it was me who had to tell them that the pregnancy was gone.

This post was terribly painful to write. It was even hard to even push the button to post. But little did I know at the time, a remarkable change in the path of my life was coming.

BEATRICE'S STORY

I also had a loss nine months after the birth of my first. I had the privilege of carrying that baby with me for those few weeks. It does not matter how much time goes by. I still feel guilt and sadness even though I know that I did not cause my miscarriage. According to my doctor, it just happens and there is not a great reason to explain it sometimes. I just hold on to my faith knowing that there is a little angel waiting for me when I go to heaven.

Join the movement. Share these stories so that we all have a voice. #TheLightAfterLoss

@siramara

Sandy Bodeau

@sanbodeau

CHAPTER 7

THEY WILL WANT TO SHOW THEIR SUPPORT

August 18, 2017

"The very same people that were happy for you will be sad with you and would want to show their support." My husband's wise words. And you all have proven him right. So many sweet messages that have me blown away. I am finding peace with each second that goes by but I'm also grieving and your words are making a beautiful difference. I'm forever grateful for you, my Instafam.

> *"You have an entire community that wants to support you and be there for you. He is so right."*
>
> *"I am so sorry for your loss. God does things for a reason. Every time you feel down or sad just carry your handsome little prince."*

"You have a community." It was such a powerful statement. With each message, it became more and more clear that there was something bigger going on. Behind those little square photos and catchy anecdotes we share in search of likes, behind the popularity game and its players, there were real people. Actual souls dealing with hurdles, pain and, like me, loss. In between my moments of grief, I began seeing glimpses of light. There was, in fact, a positive side to having been forced to publicly share that I'd had a miscarriage.

But not every comment was easy to read. To begin with, it was too early to hear that God does everything for a reason. Why would God want me suffering this way? Failure. I was a failure. Did God want me to feel like that? Clearly, people telling me that it would get better were saying that with the best intentions. But I knew they were wrong. The devastation that miscarriage leaves in you does not get better. What many people did not know was that I knew this from personal experience, having miscarried the first time a year and a half prior.

Almost everything that hurt to read was intended to help. With miscarriage, people often do not know what to say, and I understood that. It was like the comments encouraging me to just hold Lennox and look at him to find comfort. The problem was that all I felt was guilt when I looked at him during those first few days post-miscarriage. Having another child was largely so that he could have what I'd had growing up. My childhood was filled with unforgettable memories that I share with my brothers. I wanted to give him another little person to build that bond with. And I was simply failing him.

A majority of the messages were sweet and heartwarming. Nevertheless, there was an overwhelming sadness from having so many unanswered text messages from close friends and direct messages from loyal Instagram followers. How could I ever reply to them? What could I possibly say? And then there were the ones who had not heard the news about my miscarriage and were still sending their congratulations. I just read and cried.

Anyone who has faced loss knows the feeling. Whether that loss be the loss of love, loss of a loved one, or loss of a baby. The pain of loss is numbing. It is no different when you have a miscarriage. It is so hard for people to understand this pain because it is caused by the loss of someone you never got to meet. It is even hard for the woman experiencing it to understand how it can hurt so much. But it does.

At times, your arms and legs become heavy. Your stomach tightens and a sense of nausea crawls through your body. Your mind becomes numb. When you wake up each morning, the beauty of a new day is swept away by the darkness and grim reality of yesterday.

But there was something happening, and even amid the pain and sadness it was hard not to notice. When I told my husband that I could not find a way to tell everyone that I had lost my baby, we talked about how deep some of my online connections had become. He reminded me that all of these people were only wanting to support me. And they would want to show that support – not just in the excitement of the good news, but share in the reality of news that was harder to take.

We also talked about the women who had been reaching out to me. Women sharing stories of their own losses after I had shared that Lennox was a rainbow baby. I was moved by both the depth of their honesty and the number of messages I received. It was clear that I had struck a chord by opening up.

Recently, it had often been me on the other side of things. A growing number of people I follow had begun to share not just the cute outfit pictures and manicured family photos all filled with smiles, but real stories of challenges faced, and pain felt. And I, too, had found comfort in knowing I was not alone when those women spoke about their miscarriages. It was my time to share my struggles in the hope of helping others like others had done for me.

As soon as I shared this 'there is no easy way to say it' post, the outpouring commenced in volumes. It touched me deeply. There were messages of support and messages from others sharing stories of their own losses. That post marked a profound change in my life that I only vaguely began to understand at the time. Little did I know that my rushed announcement and following miscarriage would start a transformational journey that my Instagram community embraced in a very unexpected way.

DANIELA'S STORY

I grew up hearing that my mom had a loss before my older brother was born. I always knew how common miscarriage was. When I first got pregnant, I was very aware of the statistics. But the theory never resembles reality. What hurt the most after I miscarried was feeling like I was crying an illusion, a life that I imagined and was not going to happen – at least not at the moment. I felt a void in my chest from missing something that I never felt, that I never hugged, that I never … anything. It is a very lonely grief.

My relatives tried to comfort me with the typical 'everything happens for a reason' – a phrase that made me want to know more about the reason for something that I will simply never know. Now I just want other women who go through this to know that they are not alone, that everything they feel is normal, that they have the right to mourn their loss, the right to talk about this without feeling any shame, the right to cry as much as they need to. You have the right to see your friends with healthy pregnancies and feel the 'why not me?' You have the right to want to try again as soon as your doctor allows you to and you also have the right to wait as long as you need.

Join the movement. Share these stories so that we all have a voice. #TheLightAfterLoss

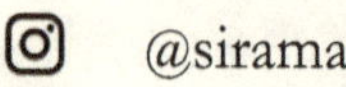

@siramara
Sandy Bodeau
@sanbodeau

CHAPTER 8

HIDING

August 20, 2017

Hide. That is all you want to do. Not having to face anyone to share the tragic news. My heart literally sinks with every buzz of my phone thinking that I have to tell yet another friend. But I have chosen not to hide. I have chosen to speak openly about it because hiding feels like you're blaming yourself even more so than the fact itself already makes you blame yourself. I lick my wounds every few minutes, I break down, and then I say it because I've learned something thanks to many of you messaging me in the last few days: we suffer in silence when this happens and suffering alone is way harder than suffering surrounded by love. #ihadamiscarriage

"Oh mama, I'm so sorry for your loss. You are so strong for sharing your life with the world. I'm sure it's helping others out there struggling. Hugs to you and your darling family."

During those days, I felt anything but strong. I felt like a broken toy. But people were sending me messages of support, and messages thanking me for my strength. And that caused me to search for the truth behind their words. Could this pain be turned into something good? Were others really benefiting from hearing that someone shared their struggle?

There I stood at a crossroads. This second miscarriage was devastating in more ways that I can count or even begin to explain. Those who have experienced a pregnancy loss, or any sort of infertility issues, will agree that it involves not just sadness of loss. The pain and sadness is tightly wrapped in guilt, self-doubt, and even self-hatred. The questions swirl in and around your mind from the moment you wake up until the moment you fall asleep, exhausted. Why did my body let me down? What did I do wrong? Could my partner ever forgive me for my failure to bring a baby into our lives? The layers of pain and anxiety are immense.

So here we were again. Pregnant one moment, not pregnant the next. But the pain of this second miscarriage was much more acute than the first. The first miscarriage had been a scare, as well as a loss. The realization that my health, perhaps even my life, had been at risk had given me an unexpected perspective. Even with the loss and the profound sadness that came with it, I felt genuinely lucky to be alive that first time. Also, it really did not hit me as hard emotionally, because I always thought that it was an isolated event.

How quickly our self-image can change. Instead of being amazed at what my body had been capable of doing just six months before – giving life and then giving birth to my son – I now felt ashamed for what it was not able to do. In just a matter of days, my perception of my powerful body had been erased.

The first miscarriage could no longer be seen as an isolated event. Not only had I lost my precious baby, but gone too was an important part of myself. What was now lost was the fearless warrior within me. The warrior I had inherited from my mother.

My mother might not be as tall as me, but from her I learned a strength, conviction and fearlessness that had driven me throughout my life. My mother endured great losses as well, losses we shared. But despite the setbacks, she retained a fierce warrior mentality. My mother is hard working, incredibly determined, and tough as nails.

In my neighborhood in Madrid, my mother was not one to trifle with. Nor would it be wise to slight any of her three children. We lived in a neighborhood with zero diversity. So, when my oldest brother was born, everyone wanted to see what a bi-racial child looked like. Unaware of why people constantly stopped her to look at the baby, my sweet Abuela just proudly showed off her first grandchild. But my mama knew why people were looking. There were ridiculous rumors about bi-racial children having white ears and a darker face and things like that. Everyone wanted a look at my brother, but never around my mom. Everyone knew she was not afraid to speak up, and the little crowds would quickly dissipate as soon as they saw her appear.

I am definitely my mother's daughter when it comes to speaking up and toughness. 'Sandra the Warrior' has always been such a natural part of my character that I took it for granted. But now, suddenly, I felt incredibly vulnerable. There was a crack in the armor of my invincibility. This body that I honed and treated like a well-oiled machine had shown its humanity. My will was not enough to bring a baby into our lives. There I was, an empty shell of myself and feeling defeated.

Throughout my pregnancy with Lennox, my optimism remained. I did not let bleeding, trips to the hospital for early contractions, gestational diabetes or intense pain dampen my resolve. My warrior spirit stayed strong and I never lost faith. And in the end, I was right not to question. The Warrior was right. All 9 ½ pounds of Lennox proved that the first miscarriage was a mirage.

But now, the mirage had reappeared. And this time it was clear that it was not a mirage at all. It was very real; real in a humbling way. Darkness cascaded around me like a heavy woolen blanket. The light I had found with Lennox – the light I had fought so hard not to lose – was fading. I kept praying to find it, but I just felt lost, confused and angry.

JULENE'S STORY

I was 27 when I got pregnant for the first time. The timing was perfect: my marriage was great and I had a good job. We got pregnant on our first try. We saw a heartbeat on the first visit to the doctor. Then, at nine weeks, I started bleeding. I took it very hard. I could not understand why this had happened to me. I thought I was the only woman in my group of friends that had ever gone through it. Turns out that, upon my sharing, several friends shared that they had also had a miscarriage. It took us a year to feel ready to try again. Sadly, history repeated itself.

I started feeling like the 'it just happens sometimes' explanation that doctors were giving me was not good enough. I was told that more extensive testing was not necessary unless you experience four losses, and I simply could not understand why I had to wait to go through two more miscarriages in order to get an answer. I found a doctor that finally agreed to do further testing, only to get results that indicated that nothing was wrong with me.

I cried night after night asking God to please allow me to carry a healthy pregnancy. We moved to another country and, in the midst of the crazy process of adapting to a new place, I got pregnant with my first daughter. She came to teach us that the best things in life happen in the most unexpected moments.

A year after having my first daughter, we decided to try to get pregnant again and did so on the first try. Shockingly, I miscarried again. Why did this keep happening to me? I decided to find a specialist and finally got a diagnosis: antiphospholipid syndrome. I started to get treated right away and got pregnant shortly after. Another miscarriage. The most traumatic one, as I had to get two D&Cs (after the first one failed to extract all the tissue). I decided to stop trying to look for answers. I had a daughter to take care of. But, deep in my heart, I kept asking God to allow me to give my child a sibling.

And, just like it happened with my first daughter, I got pregnant after we moved to another country and when we were least expecting it. My second daughter came to tell me that nothing is as we planned, that we just need to let go and open our heart to what life may have in store for us.

Join the movement. Share these stories so that we all have a voice. #TheLightAfterLoss

@siramara
Sandy Bodeau
@sanbodeau

CHAPTER 9

TURN IT INTO A LESSON

August 22, 2017

A week ago at this time, I was pregnant. Five hours later, I wasn't anymore. A friend told me today: "I admire how you turn everything into a lesson." I am not sure that I see the lesson yet but I know that I'll be stronger once the hardest part of this storm passes. After several days of not dressing myself, I decided to try some gorgeous clothes by my @lapontedesigner to remind myself of how much I love my job and how fortunate I am to have friends to work with. #ihadamiscarriage

> *"I'm blown away by your honesty. I'm so sorry, my dear. God bless you. All will be well again in time."*

Was that the lesson I needed to learn from this very public miscarriage? Was my honesty a vehicle towards helping others feel less isolated? It was precisely because I had always tried to turn everything into a lesson that I knew how hard it was to do. It is always easier to sit down and dwell on your reality. It is easier to feel sorry for yourself. Actually, it is also necessary. But not forever. And it was time for me to begin to find my lesson.

There was definitely a growing sense that something had changed. And it was not simply the loss of a child and a future reality that had already been taking shape in my mind. The pain and the heaviness never left, but I was taking note of the power of human connection in the era of social media.

The outpouring remained constant. Every single day, women I had never met were reaching out to me and sharing their stories. This was shockingly unexpected. They were opening up, many for the first time to anyone. Each message I read brought tears to my eyes, knowing exactly what they meant when they said: "I know you will understand." My head nodded and tears flowed as I read those words. Of course I understood.

Each message was answered as if a close friend had sent it to me. As they read my replies, I was sure that they were also reading with tears in their eyes. We had connected as part of a sisterhood we did not want to be part of. But we were all finding comfort in realizing that we were not the only member of the group. We were not alone. There were others just like us.

Even though I did not know any of the women opening their hearts to me in such a raw way, the bond I felt with them was closer than I felt with anyone else around me. And that is why they were choosing to tell me. Just like when I read their messages, they knew that I understood in a way that no one else could.

Those messages made me reflect on what someone else had commented a few days before. My social media presence was turning away from being a way to share my professional experiences (first my jewelry business then my blogging and TV adventures). It was becoming a community of women who were connecting with me at a very intimate level. And so it was that only days after my second miscarriage, I began to see that my loss could be turned into a lesson. I began to find a purpose.

Compassion was the primary feeling I had for those who chose to share their own loss with me. But I was also very grateful. We were each walking the same path, but I was in a powerful position, a privileged one.

The thousands of people who joined my Instagram community for fashion tips were now listening and engaging. They were connecting with me about a prevalent issue among women that almost no one was willing to talk about.

Suddenly, I felt a duty to continue to be honest with them. No longer would I contribute to the perpetuation of the stigma and taboo associated with miscarriage. This may not have been the path I chose, but it was my path. And it was becoming obvious that I was walking it for a reason.

In spite of the darkness all around me, or perhaps because of it, those women were showing me a light. Unable to find my own path to overcome the tremendous pain, the willingness of others to share their story with me was leading me towards a very powerful path.

Like I had done many times before, including moving to another country by myself with only $800, I decided to take a leap of faith and go where this new light was taking me. There was a profound feeling that something bigger than me, my experience and my voice would be found by following the light that each one of these women were showing me. My friend was right. This miscarriage was going to lead me to one of my greatest lessons.

VANESSA'S STORY

I have never talked about this with anybody other than my husband. Not even my mother knows. I have had three miscarriages from natural pregnancies. I finally decided to try IVF, as I felt that there had to be something wrong with me even though I was never diagnosed for my infertility issues. It took us four years to get pregnant, even with IVF. I thought that I would never get to be a mother.

I wish I would have had the courage to share my story in the way you are sharing it. Even now that I already have my rainbow baby, I find comfort in your words. And I am sure that I am not alone. You are making me realize that all those years of struggle when I felt completely alone, there were probably women around me going through the same.

Feeling like it is only happening to you is awful. I wish I would have said something but I was so ashamed. I went through so many emotions, and I am not sure that I will ever forget them. I was angry and I felt guilty because my body was not doing what it was naturally designed to do as a woman: create life. Those three miscarriages still hurt, and your honesty is helping me feel understood.

———————

Join the movement. Share these stories so that we all have a voice. #TheLightAfterLoss

  @siramara

  Sandy Bodeau

  @sanbodeau

CHAPTER 10

YOU CAN BE BOTH

August 24, 2017

You can be both. You can be shocked and hurt and still be happy. You can still enjoy the many blessings in your life and not give two f#^% about what anyone thinks about your grieving process. My husband knows how I grieve when he holds me at night when I cry. My mama knows how I grieve when she takes care of my son so I can just have a bad moment. And in between all of those, I AM HAPPY. #ihadamiscarriage

"Everyone grieves differently. No one should judge. Live your life the way you see fit. You have to be strong for your son, who depends on you. If you're happy, he's happy (and his smile says it all)! I like your positive attitude! #BeHappy!"

Only a few days after my miscarriage, I started to feel glimpses of joy. We decided to go to the beach – my happy place – for the first time after my miscarriage. Life flowed back into me as we began walking on the sand. The breeze, the sun, the waves. All those elements have always been such contributors to a magnificent feeling of peace. Immediately, I wanted my husband to capture the moment. I wanted to look back at that picture in order to remember that there would be moments that I felt happiness in spite of my heartbreak.

Coincidentally, I was carrying a Peace, Love, World towel that said, "I am happy." So I decided to lay on my towel purposefully showing the message and my husband snapped a picture. When he handed me the phone so I could see the shots, doubt crept in. Should I share the picture, looking happy and relaxed?

There was nothing wrong with the picture, but I knew where my doubts were coming from. Just days after announcing my second miscarriage, the picture did not show me looking sad. That left me angry with myself and my contradictory feelings. One minute excited to feel like myself again, the next punishing myself for not looking sad enough.

Sitting down on the towel, I took a deep breath and wrote the above post. It was good to be happy. We all grieve differently. The fact that I had found joy in a place with such a strong link to my peace and happiness did not take away the fact that I was still heartbroken.

Not only that, as my follower's comment stated very well, we all need happiness. My six-month-old baby did not need to learn anything about grief yet. In that moment, I vowed to never again feel guilt for not being in a constant state of grief. Just as an athlete can manage to finish a race even with an injured foot, I was going to let happiness into my life even with a broken heart.

That is one of life's important lessons that I was re-learning. We can never assume how someone is feeling based on their behavior. The cheeriest person could be facing a tremendous battle. Maybe that good attitude was exactly what she needed in order to pull herself out of darkness. Or it may simply be their way of keeping up their guard to avoid being asked what is wrong. Similarly, someone with a bad attitude could simply be having a stressful day or have received bad news minutes before your encounter. None of those reactions define that individual as a person. Those small moments really do not say much about who we are.

This entire experience was also revealing a lot about my relationship with my husband. The start of it had been a whirlwind and we were crazy in love. Things moved so quickly for us. We had not faced any challenge as a couple until we faced the loss of our first child. In less than two years, we had now lost two very wanted babies.

Thankfully, that heartbreak gave us the opportunity to learn what our relationship was made of. Laying in his arms with my head on his chest, I cried myself to sleep more times than I can count. In between my sobs, I could hear his heart. This brought me so much peace. And it reminded me of the early stages of our relationship when hearing his heartbeat was my very own sound machine to help me fall asleep at night.

This miscarriage provided another opportunity. It helped me build an even stronger bond with my mom. While I felt blessed for it, I wished that she had not had to see me go through such dark times. During the first miscarriage, she had helped me from a distance. But she was visiting when the second miscarriage happened and she was immersed in my suffering. Seeing her own child in such pain was extremely difficult for her. It was through watching me in tears so many times that she finally understood that you are not any weaker when you cry.

My mom is the toughest person that I know. Her first reaction to watching one of her children visibly upset had always been to say, "Don't cry." Amidst the pain of this miscarriage, I asked her why she always said that. Crying was what my mind and body needed and no one needed to tell me that I should not. She confessed that it was just too painful for her to see me crying. But hearing her own words, she understood that she needed to put my suffering first and simply let me cry.

My mother learned that lesson, and I also learned something. Clearly, I was not the only one suffering. Even though I felt that no one could understand the pain I was going through, my family was also suffering with me and for me. The pain and fear that accompanies miscarriage goes way beyond the person who physically goes through it and her partner. Many of our loved ones are also scarred by it.

And though I was seeing glimpses of strength and happiness, we all had a long road ahead.

SHANNON'S STORY

My sister and I are four years apart because my mom had several miscarriages during that time. I don't know how she coped. She had two more babies after all that loss. I pulled eight eggs during my IVF egg retrieval and only one embryo survived. I thought to myself that that could have been seven miscarriages if I had gone the natural route. Such devastation and despair crippled me as I pinned all my hopes on one tiny embryo. I share this because it is important to know you are not alone and there is understanding and empathy out there as well as sympathy for your loss.

Join the movement. Share these stories so that we all have a voice. #TheLightAfterLoss

@siramara

Sandy Bodeau

@sanbodeau

CHAPTER 11

ROLLER COASTER

September 2, 2017

It has been a roller coaster of emotions since #ihadamiscarriage three weeks ago but look at these bright eyes. My son. My legacy. My reason to work harder and harder every day to be a better human. That light in those eyes will forever keep me strong. #LennoxRyan

"As a mom who has lost two, I can relate to the pain you've gone through. Much love to you. Your son is lucky to have such a wonderful mama!"

Someone who relates to your pain. That is all we want while going through any kind of hardship. As humans, we have a need to feel connected, no matter how independent we think we are. For weeks, I felt an immeasurable amount of guilt each time I held Lennox. Now, I was finally able to fully reconnect with my beautiful boy.

Yes, he was a lucky boy. My love for him was so big that I was willing to keep trying to give him a younger sibling. The love that I felt when I looked into those bright eyes would give me the necessary strength to try again. My heart was still bleeding from my latest loss, but I knew I was going to keep trying for him.

Just three days before, my friend Anabelle Blum invited me to participate in a photo shoot for her line of t-shirts. Her line focused on women's empowerment, and she had chosen me to be the image of her 'Super Mom' t-shirt. With my 7-month-old baby on my hip, the photographer took the pictures. Beautiful makeup. Gorgeous hairstyle.

Powerful t-shirt. My always-smiley baby by my side. Back at work just two weeks after my miscarriage. Yes, I felt like a super mom.

But I also felt like an impostor. Like someone who was just pretending to have it all together. In reality, I had been doing nothing but doubt my strength for the last few weeks. Those are thoughts I try to kick to the curb, to the best of my ability. So I decided to enjoy the photo shoot and give myself some credit. Maybe I did not feel as powerful as the t-shirt showed, but I was strong enough to push through. Pushing through is the first step towards doing better, and there is a power in that as well.

Once my part of the shoot was done, I sat down for a few minutes to get something to eat. One of the women from the shoot approached me and said: "Next time you get pregnant, do not say anything to anyone. There are many people out there who love you, but there are also people out there who do not want to see you doing well." It was not ill intended. It was said by a woman who loves me. But, in a matter of seconds, this woman's words sent me right back into a dark hole.

Only recently had I begun to work through the immense guilt I felt for convincing my husband to go public with our pregnancy before he was ready. He was still receiving congratulatory messages. And now, someone was telling me how irresponsible I had been for making my announcement too early. Not only that, she was also telling me that it had been the negative energy that I attracted to our life that had caused my miscarriage. That is not what she meant, but that is exactly what I heard then.

Earlier that day, I walked into the room feeling energized. But now I left the place absolutely deflated. I called my brother Manu, tears running down my face, asking if he thought that I was attracting bad energy and that is why I had miscarried. As he always does, he comforted me and told me to stop listening to what anyone had to say and focus on my healing.

Doing my best to try to follow my brother's advice, I decided to go to an album release party that night. My hair and makeup were still done from the shoot, so I was going to make the most of it. It was also the kind of event that would be great for a girl hiding her emotions to go to. It would be loud and impossible to even hear any hurtful comment that may have come my way.

It was a great event and I actually enjoyed myself. It was good to be surrounded by a positive atmosphere, talk about simple things and be dressed up for the first time in weeks. I was still struggling, but I was slowly rebuilding my strength.

Just three days after that, we received some devastating news. My father-in-law had passed away. It happened as we debated whether to evacuate our house due to the threat of Hurricane Irma coming directly toward Miami. Obviously, that took care of our evacuation decision. We rented a van, packed it with family, pets and important belongings, and headed to West Virginia so my husband could say his last goodbye to his father.

A tragic occurrence, but one that was oddly therapeutic. Immediately, I went into caregiver mode, completely forgetting all the feelings that I had been having during the last few weeks. Taking care of my husband became my priority. My focus was on making sure that he felt supported and loved.

The loss of a father was something I knew all too well, and my heart was breaking for him. The chaos that surrounded us during those days – between the hurricane and the loss of my father-in-law – quickly snapped me out of the darkness. I had a family to take care of, and that is what I was going to do.

NADIA'S STORY

I lost my baby almost six months into the pregnancy. I had to deliver him. It happened due to chorioamnionitis. This is an infection in the urinary tract. The guilt is killing me. I carried the infection, so this is my fault. I was going to do IVF next, but the loss sent me into a terrible depression and I just don't feel ready. I do not know if I ever will. Believe it or not, in the middle of my mourning process, I still think that life is beautiful and I am thankful for people like you choosing to speak up about these issues and give those of us who are suffering in silence a voice.

Join the movement. Share these stories so that we all have a voice. #TheLightAfterLoss

@siramara

Sandy Bodeau

@sanbodeau

CHAPTER 12

AFTER THE STORM

September 14, 2017

In the last month, we've lost a parent, a baby and faced the possibility of losing our home due to #HurricaneIrma (thank you God for that miracle). I have learned

1. That sending a parent to heaven without unresolved issues and lots of love is what every child deserves

2. That I am in absolute control of my emotions and finding peace within sadness is healthy and necessary

3. That I care about material things less than I ever did since becoming a mother. Getting my child to a safe place was my priority and, while I was stressed out about our house, I found peace in knowing that I can overcome anything as long as my family is OK

Cheers to the best Thursday yet, my darlings!

> *"Amen! Every day we walk on this earth is a blessing. We cannot control anything in life but our own thoughts, emotions, and behavior. When you understand that and accept that, peace comes. Worry is the thief of joy. Much love to you and your family."*

The past two weeks had been a whirlwind. Irma had missed us, unlike many of our fellow Floridians, but we felt like we had weathered the storm. The drive was slow as we were joined by thousands evacuating Florida into Georgia and the Carolinas. We arrived at my father-in-law's viewing the night before the funeral. The trip had taken 36 hours, broken up by only six hours of sleep in a horrible motel we were lucky to find.

My husband is from a big family. Many of his siblings were also making the journey from other Florida cities. All of us were part of this massive pilgrimage as we went to pay respect to his father, who had been losing his battle with Alzheimer's. It had been clear for months that he was not improving. Fortunately, we had spent some nice time with him the year before.

My husband's stepmother had been admitted to the hospital. There was a shared concern that his father could not stay alone given his deteriorating condition. So eight months pregnant, I gave my husband my blessing (and encouragement) to go and bring his father to our home. That was December 23, when he made another pilgrimage of sorts. My husband made the 2000 mile journey there and back, in time for us to spend Christmas together. At least the one hour that remained.

It would have made me happy to have met my father-in-law when he had his full faculties, but he was still a warm and kind man. My husband shared that he had spent a life making mistakes, and often running away from them. He had not had a drink for many years, but that alcohol had led him to make bad decisions. It was hard for me to see anything other than the kind man I had met, but it seemed there were hard things he'd had to face and apologies to be made.

My husband always seemed at peace with his relationship with his father, even if it was limited by time and distance. He described years of his father facing his adult children, asking their forgiveness, and generally making himself available for them to work through the pains caused in large part by his general lack of availability.

His time with us was wonderful. I will never forget the patience and compassion my husband showed towards his father during those last few days they spent together. His father began each day confused by why he was at our house, why his wife was not there with him, and really just where he was in general. Each day he learned the exciting news, as if for the first time, that I was pregnant with another grandchild. It was not a simple visit, but it was rewarding. And I saw that my husband was at peace with their relationship. It made me happy that his father's visit had provided my husband with any closure that he may have still needed.

My father-in-law spent similar time with each of my husband's siblings. Each had a similar experience. My husband was glad that the visit gave some of his siblings the closure that they perhaps had not found fully in the years prior. It seemed to have been a blessing for all of them. That meant that we were a part of a unique experience when we paid our last respects. It is not often that children are able to say their last respects without harboring unresolved issues. But here we were, celebrating life with a group of children who had their closure. It was beautiful.

By the accounts of his children, here was a man who could have left a legacy of neglect and pain that could have lingered for generations. Instead, his willingness to face his fears and demons left his children with a blessing. Peace.

I remember holding my husband's hand as he saw his father for the last time, and I saw peace within his sadness. It made me reflect about the other journey of loss we had been going through for the last few weeks. I had also found peace within my sadness. But, unlike my husband, there had been no closure for me.

There was no one to blame but myself for the demons still haunting me after my miscarriages. There was no one to make amends with me and help me feel better. There was no place for me to go to say a symbolic last goodbye to the pain I was carrying with me. But, like my father-in-law, I was ready to face my fears and take control of the situation. Deep in my heart, I knew that my answers would come one day.

JENNIFER'S STORY

Like you, I also know what it feels to have a miscarriage. It was 10 years ago. I know it sounds like a long time ago, but it still feels as if it happened yesterday.

Like any woman who has been praying to get pregnant, I was elated when I learned that a baby boy was going to join our family. He was so wanted. And then he was gone before we even got to meet him.

I still wonder why I hid. Why I have stayed silent for all these years. Why almost nobody is willing to talk about this. I know I am not alone. But I felt alone. I felt that nobody would understand my pain.

Join the movement. Share these stories so that we all have a voice. #TheLightAfterLoss

- @siramara
- Sandy Bodeau
- @sanbodeau

CHAPTER 13

COUNTING BLESSINGS

May 5, 2018

He's given me the best days of my life and I want to give him the best life. I was talking to a dear friend about the not so easy road to baby #2 and I realized that I already got my biggest blessing by having my #LennoxRyan. I'm gonna keep the faith and think that whatever will be, will be and, in the interim, I'll enjoy every second like this like they will not come back – because they are not.

"Sending you guys alllll the love! You are so blessed to have each other."

The conversation mentioned above was with my friend Lindsey. Her second child was born weeks apart from what would have been the birth of my second child. I somewhat embarrassingly confessed to her that it was painful for me to watch her precious little boy because, by watching him, I knew exactly how old mine would have been. She was incredibly supportive and understanding. It felt good to say those words out loud instead of silently suffering.

That taught me that my feelings were valid and nothing to be ashamed of. You have the right to feel sad and you can tell the people around you how you feel. Not only can you, but in fact you should. The people who love you will want to know about your struggles and will offer comfort. No one knows what you are going through after a miscarriage unless you tell them. Eight months after my loss, probably no one thought that the pain was still lingering and that I was still being hurt by what I saw around me.

Unlike after my first miscarriage, we had decided to take some time before trying again to get pregnant. There was a lot of healing that needed to happen. The second miscarriage was shocking and absolutely unexpected. It was a reminder that it could happen again, something I never considered possible after my first loss. So, we waited.

We waited about four months to try again. We had always become pregnant very easily. But, unlike my previous pregnancies, it was not happening as quickly this time. That made me begin to question whether getting pregnant again would happen at all. I was becoming a woman I did not want to be. Whenever someone else announced a pregnancy, I felt sadness. And I knew exactly who was pregnant at the same time that I had been, like Lindsey. My head hurt and I felt out of breath each time one of those women posted a picture of a baby being born when mine would have been.

There was also a growing awareness within me that the pain of women like me was a pain that is diminished by society. The loss of a child is not considered as sympathetic if that woman has another child. Whenever someone said how blessed I was to have Lennox, it felt like they were adding "so get over it" at the end.

Yes, I was blessed to have Lennox. He was my pride and joy and I felt fortunate to be his mom daily. But having him did not take away the pain that not being able to complete our family brought into my life. In my heart, I knew our family needed another member, and I was unable to fulfill that. As a woman, probably because you are the carrier of that life, you feel a much bigger duty to your family to take care of that. So I began to put so much pressure on myself and became terrified of the possibility of never being able to carry a pregnancy to term again.

It takes a lot of personal growth, pain and tears to understand that you are not failing. I wish I could tell you that you immediately feel that way, but I would not be being honest with you. It is a process. Working out and eating well were conscious decisions to treat my body with care and to make it a proper vessel to carry another child. But Mother Nature seemed to scoff at this, and I hated her often for failing to fulfill her end of the bargain.

Almost daily, I doubted myself and my abilities to overcome hurdles — which I had rarely doubted before — due to my failed attempts to add to our family. In order to conquer your infertility process, you are going to walk that path. It is the path of doubt and sadness that will hopefully lead you to acceptance. Like everything else in life, all we can do is try our best. Once you know you have done all that you can, you must stop punishing yourself.

After speaking to Lindsey and others, I was on my way to learning how to stop punishing myself. Talking about my feelings with others was one of the first steps. That required self-awareness and a recognition that I struggled with my feelings. Many times, I was not proud of those feelings. But I wanted this journey to make me a better person and not a bitter one.

It was ironic that just as I was having those conversations for the first time and letting people know that I had doubts about being able to carry another baby, Mother Nature had a surprise in store for me. I was pregnant for the fourth time without even knowing it. But it was not the only surprise.

CARRIE'S STORY

Product of Conception. That is what they called him. Sterile words spoken in a sterile hospital room by oblivious technicians about my dead baby. No one stopped to look me in the eye. No one saw me. No one saw him. There were no sympathies or condolences just procedure and protocol. After four weeks of my body refusing to let go of the baby that was still inside of me, I was admitted for a dilation and curettage procedure, a D&C.

After hours of waiting in agony, a hurried nurse began the pre-operative interview. Never looking up, she indifferently noted my answers. "How many live births have you had?" she eventually asked, as she procedurally worked her way down the long list of standard questions.

"Eight."

She stopped taking notes for a second and glanced sideway in my direction. "Honey, you have eight children?"

"No," I began. "I have 10 children. Eight on earth and two in heaven." A lump settled in my throat and hot tears sprung to my eyes. "Each one of them is a precious gift."

The nurse hesitated a second and then softened and offered a sympathetic smile before she resumed her long litany of sterile questions.

For a second his life was acknowledged. For a tiny second he was more than a product of conception, he was a person. A person that is deeply missed. A person that in the mere moments of his existence is pure gift. A little soul with a name. We call him Michael.

CHAPTER 14

MY OWN STRENGTH

May 24, 2018

Have been listening non-stop to Whitney Houston's 'I Didn't Know My Own Strength'. Powerful.

'I love you' — Anabelle

Another cryptic message and a supportive response from a close friend. Anabelle was among the very small group of people who knew that I had miscarried again.

On May 17th, I found out that I was pregnant. And on May 24th I miscarried again. After eight months of hoping that it would happen for us again (though just four months really trying), hope had come but was gone again in just seven days. By the time we made it to my doctor's appointment, I was no longer pregnant.

My doctor came into the room. It was a scene I will never forget. We had previously called her to let her know that I was bleeding, so she knew the chances were that I had miscarried again. She looked at me with a somber face and asked: "What happened?" I looked down, mortified. Ashamed of myself. What was the answer to her question? I had no idea! I was so angry and disappointed. I wanted to scream: "MY BODY HAS BETRAYED ME AGAIN!!! THAT IS WHAT HAPPENED!"

In between tears, I asked my husband to tell her what had happened the previous days. He explained that we had taken several pregnancy tests and that all of them had come back positive but with very faint lines. That seemed to indicate that my hCG levels had been low from the get-go. We noticed those very light lines, but simply assumed that it was because it was super early in the pregnancy. My doctor ordered some tests to confirm that I was no longer pregnant. We left her office; I do not think that I ever looked up again after her question.

I kept Whitney Houston's 'I Didn't Know My Own Strength' on repeat and played it no matter where I was. The lyrics were so powerful. She and I rekindled the bond we had formed, when as a young woman, I would channel my inner-Whitney in karaoke bars throughout Madrid. The lyrics describe her battles with the demons that led her to substance abuse. Our battles were different, but we had both learned that searching for your own strength was the answer to winning the war, battle by battle. And, yes, I was going through my darkest hours.

Once again, I had to pick myself back up. Holding my head up high was becoming harder than the last time, but I had begun to understand that I needed to do so. Little by little, I began giving myself more grace.

After this third loss, I found a different kind of strength. The strength was a welcomed surprise, but I worried a bit about where it came from. Maybe it was because I had barely had time to even get excited that I was pregnant. But maybe I was just getting used to terrible news. That was something I feared. Pain is needed in order to truly overcome adversity, so I did not want to become immune to it. To become numb. The kind of numbness that does not allow you to feel anything, good or bad.

As crazy as it may sound, I made a conscious decision to immerse myself in my pain this time. This was not a fight I could win, so I was going to make the pain my ally. In order to pick myself up, I had to be willing to go head first into the dark hole that this infertility journey had sent me on. It was a painful journey, but it was my journey.

This pain was no longer going to be the captain of my life's journey. I was going to lead. As captain, I would find out how to use this pain as fuel.

With the clarity that perspective gives you, I encourage those of you who face pregnancy loss to do the same. You cannot make the pain disappear. It is going to hurt. But you can learn about it. You can walk with it hand in hand as partners. Because that pain becomes part of your life after a miscarriage. You will never remember the miscarriage without pain. Welcome it into your life as an opportunity to become stronger. And to do so, you just have to let it in. Learn from it. Embrace it for what it is. It is a part of your journey.

What you must do is to fight the numbness that comes with the loss. You must not partner with the numbness. You need to FEEL. Do not be afraid of feeling that pain. Believe me, like Whitney beautifully sang, you will be surprised by your own strength.

ADRIANA'S STORY

I have just been told that I lost my baby. Other than the father, you are the first person I am sharing this with. I think nobody else will understand me unless they have gone through it.

We had not told anybody about the pregnancy. We wanted to wait until our first ultrasound. Just yesterday, they told me everything was OK, and today my baby is gone. I have no idea how I will face the day tomorrow. The only good part is that I have my 2-year-old to keep me strong. I know you know the feeling. But I still feel terrible. This little heartbeat stopped at six weeks of pregnancy.

We moved to a new house during that week and I had to go to Amsterdam for a work trip. I am convinced that this is my fault and that I could have avoided this miscarriage. The stress of that week was what caused this loss. Getting over the guilt I feel for not having done things differently will be the hardest obstacle to overcome for me.

———————

Join the movement. Share these stories so that we all have a voice. #TheLightAfterLoss

@siramara

Sandy Bodeau

@sanbodeau

CHAPTER 15

ANOTHER SUCCESSFUL MISCARRIAGE

June 8, 2018

"YOU HAVE SUCCESSFULLY COMPLETED YOUR MISCARRIAGE" {5/29/18}. I dropped my phone. I knew I was having another miscarriage – my third – but I had no idea that there was anything 'successful' about losing a baby.

You are left with so many questions and, not going to lie, anger. I was angry at my body. A body I nurture daily had failed me. Again. I knew I needed to give myself some time to grieve & feel those feelings (hence my TV break and not attending fashion week).

But as soon as those two weeks were over, I went back to who I am: someone who turns negatives into positives. I know that I've been given this journey for a reason. Perhaps because I am outspoken and feel a responsibility to not hide the pain that miscarriages come with? I don't have the answer today, but I know that I am walking this path so others don't walk it alone. I am here. I know how you feel. I did not expect it, but here I am. And I'm going to be a better human because of it. Fertility issues have chosen me but I am choosing to turn them into a super power. #UnfilteredMamasClub

"God will give you the strength you need to overcome this new test, Sandy. I admire so much how you are facing these challenges. How you are managing to turn your sadness into strength for others. Not all of us would be able to do so. You receive what you give. God's timing is perfect. You will be rewarded for

your beautiful heart and for how much of it you are willing to share so others feel less alone. Sending you so much love!"

'Success' is defined as 'the accomplishment of an aim or purpose.' How could someone tell me that, by losing a third child, I had accomplished any kind of purpose? Medically speaking, those words meant that I had done a good job at passing all the tissue that remained in my body once I lost my baby. But that choice of words felt all sorts of wrong.

There was something, however, that felt all sorts of right. It was reading the comments and messages that kept coming from my dear Instagram community. It confirmed that there were women out there who needed to read what I had to say about my experience with miscarriage. Out of the darkness I was finding a voice to help others feel understood and less lonely during the loneliest journey a woman can go on.

It was during the first few weeks after my third miscarriage that I truly realized my success. It was the creation of light out of darkness. There was success in this episode of my life. And it had nothing to do with my physical 'abilities' to eliminate the remains of a pregnancy we were praying for. My success was coming from having found a way to show others a path towards their own healing. A way to cope. A friend to listen when they felt like no one could understand what they were going through. That was my success after this third loss.

Looking back at the posts that followed the confession that I had lost another child, it revealed that I was taking a different approach. The focus was not on talking about my miscarriage during the weeks that followed it. And not because I did not care. Nothing could be further from the truth. Simply, I had finally been able to find strength in this fight. And I wanted those who were suddenly listening to this new voice of mine to know that

I was getting stronger. They needed to know that they could get stronger, too.

It was my duty to help them. Those women were depositing such trust in me during their dark hours. A new fire burned within me that led towards becoming an advocate for the many women struggling to conceive or to carry pregnancies to term. It was clear that many could relate to my pain and my struggles. But I not only wanted them to relate to the pain. I also wanted them to relate to the opportunity to grow that I was finally able to see.

My Instagram community had seen me evolve from business owner, to fashion blogger, to TV personality, all while sharing the fact that I had arrived in the U.S. with almost no money, no contacts, and no higher education. It is a story I often share so that others can see that extraordinary things can be achieved by ordinary people who believe in themselves. And my followers were vested in that part of my journey. So, by the time my fertility struggles came into play, my followers already felt like they had connected with me on a much more personal level. And I was determined to use that connection to help them connect with a much bigger life lesson: You can find light after loss.

DIANA'S STORY

Only my husband and two close friends know about my miscarriage. And now you. We have not shared it with anybody else. But I needed to tell someone. It lifted a huge weight off my shoulders when I shared it. It should not be considered a taboo.

What needs to happen is that our families need to stop assuming that nothing is wrong. They need to stop asking how come we are not pregnant yet. They just need to show support. Be encouraging along the healing process and also support you if you decide not to try to get pregnant again. I did not feel like I would have received that kind of support. That is why I remained silent with my family.

Join the movement. Share these stories so that we all have a voice. #TheLightAfterLoss

⃝ @siramara

f Sandy Bodeau

▸ @sanbodeau

CHAPTER 16

YOU CHOOSE YOU

June 10, 2018

**You choose who you become in the face of adversity. It either
destroys you or builds you
You can get there faster or just become a MASTER
You can dream of improvement or you can lead a MOVEMENT
You can be a worrier or just become a WARRIOR**

**#miscarriageawareness
#WHPShapes
#SANday**

"You were born a warrior and it shows daily."

My 'Sandra the Warrior' spirit was returning. My purpose was becoming clear. The lessons I had learned about myself and others through my three miscarriages could be turned into a tool to serve my social media community.

It is my belief that healing comes from turning pain into a lesson, and ideally, into a purpose. And my greatest purpose for writing this book and digging through my wounds is to help you find your purpose and share lessons we can all use to help others deal with a loss. That is true whether you have experienced miscarriage yourself or if you have a friend or loved one to help through theirs and do not even know where to start.

The lessons that we learn during our struggles should always be shared with others. What would be the value of a lesson if you simply kept it to yourself? There is a lot of power in serving others and giving purpose to a painful journey.

But you also need to know that you do not need to be a warrior every single day when you are turning pain into purpose. It was encouraging to hear this woman call me a warrior. But I do not ever want to pretend that I felt strong daily. I did not. Even after having found lots of strength in what I was doing with my struggles, there were plenty of moments when I still felt defeated and very angry at my body.

The key is to not let those moments dominate your life, because they are also necessary. You will exhaust yourself very quickly if you are constantly fighting without surrendering to those feelings at times. Trust me, this is a long distance race. If you are sprinting all the time, you will not make it to the finish line.

The finish line. We use that word as if it is an actual location that we can identify. But not only can we not identify the finish line, or when we will reach it, it is likely to change for all of us along the way.

What the finish line is will be different for each woman after miscarriage. For some, it may mean being able to carry a child. For others may mean adoption. For others, it may mean stopping trying to conceive and finding peace in that decision. Whatever the finish line is, there will be a lot of soul searching along the way. And that does not happen while you are fighting. That happens when you allow yourself to experience whatever feelings your miscarriage brought into your life. Embrace that part of the process as well.

One of the best things my multiple miscarriages taught me was to focus on simplicity. Life is not only made of peaks and valleys. Life is actually made, predominantly, of all the points you visit in between the peaks and valleys. Those really simple moments and events that fill your days can be magical if you simply take the time to feel them and stop chasing the high points.

This new focus on simplicity was evident in what I decided to share on social media during the weeks that followed. Simple beach and park visits with my boy. Cherished first times at places that brought us a peaceful joy. We were simply living life and it felt good.

But there was a different kind of post on June 23, a month after my third miscarriage. On that day, my husband, Lennox and I were part of a protest against the separation of immigrant families in the U.S. There, I bumped into my friend and MSNBC correspondent Mariana Atencio. She had been reporting on the brutal separation of children from their families as they tried to cross the U.S./Mexico border for months.

What I shared publicly was how terrible I thought it was that this was happening in this country, a country I love very much. I shared how fortunate I know that my child is and how I was simply devastated thinking that many kids are not as lucky as he is.

But I did not share one other very important realization. My friend Mariana was not simply reporting. She was giving those families a face and a voice. I watched her report from the Homestead Temporary Shelter for Unaccompanied Children in absolute awe of what she was doing. She was not simply working. She had also found a purpose in what she did for a living. And it showed in every passionate word she shared in front of her audience. An audience that could relate to her being the one talking so passionately about immigration, since she was an immigrant herself.

I had to hold back tears as I held my own child during the protest. All the while looking at the walls that contained other children who had not been held by their parents for weeks, perhaps months. Mariana was giving them a voice that many people were listening to.

Watching my friend turn her job into a purpose affirmed my growing belief that I could do that by sharing my journey to try to have a second child. I could be a voice for women facing similar struggles. In fact, the choice was made then. My purpose was to turn a painful journey into a powerful voice.

ELLE'S STORY

I have loved how you are sharing your journey, Sandy. I suffered a stillbirth 19 years ago after three consecutive miscarriages. Then, there was not a platform for me to share my grief, struggles and triumphs. At times, I do not like social media. However, it has truly been an honor to be exposed to your raw emotions and brutal honesty. It has been so many years since I faced those same struggles, and your words still resonate with me as if it had happened yesterday. I am so grateful to witness what you have decided to do with your story and wish you nothing but love and light.

Join the movement. Share these stories so that we all have a voice. #TheLightAfterLoss

@siramara

Sandy Bodeau

@sanbodeau

CHAPTER 17

IT WAS OUR SECRET

August 14, 2018

For three months, it was our secret. Only a very small group of people knew. I had become so guarded about it after multiple losses. So it was our secret.

We planned to tell everybody – as in 'real life' everybody not just social media everybody – the very day (today) that I had to have surgery to remove the remains of another pregnancy that did not go as our hearts were hoping.

I truly thought about just keeping 'our secret' a secret forever and then I got a DM that said: "I really hope that this doesn't mean that you had another miscarriage but if you did, please know that your honesty has helped me so much during my own healing process."

So, here I am. Heartbroken. But, once again, being reminded that hiding is not what I need to do because I need to give this horrendous pain some purpose.

I have no idea why this is my path but I do know that I want it to be significant.

To the person who sent me that DM: THANK YOU. Thank you for now being the one helping me during my healing process. That is what life is all about.

"WOW. I am crying. Thank you for being so honest and open about the good and the tough."

We found out I was pregnant again before I even got my cycle back after my third miscarriage. My third miscarriage literally happened just a month before this latest pregnancy. It did not even cross my mind that I could get pregnant.

Happiness was not my first reaction. Instead, I was shocked, confused, and more than a little scared. The joy from seeing a positive pregnancy test result no longer existed. That had been stolen from me over the course of my journey. It was a realization that wore very heavy in my heart. That was the reason for the silence this time around. After all of the pain from my journey, and the recent miscarriage that I had had no time to come to grips with, I was not ready to go on another roller coaster ride publicly.

It felt like the right decision to simply enjoy the news in private. We literally told just three people: my mom and my two brothers. And they were sworn to secrecy. The words of the woman who told me that I had attracted bad energy into my pregnancies were still resonating in my head. Today, I know that I did nothing to cause my miscarriages. But at the time, the fear still had a place in my mind. And I let it affect me more than I should have.

Please, learn from me. Do not let anyone make you feel like anything you did was the cause of your miscarriage. There will be tons of people with great intentions saying really unfortunate things. Do yourself a favor and block out that noise while you focus on your healing.

That is what I decided to do after I learned about this fourth miscarriage. It was my fifth pregnancy. My third miscarriage after having Lennox. Try as I did to stay positive, I was losing that fight. Having gone through so much loss in such a short period of time made it almost impossible to see beyond the darkness.

In the days prior to this second doctor's visit, my body felt different. I had gone from being nauseous all day long to feeling perfectly fine. Maybe I had just gone through the nausea stage, I told myself. But deep in my heart, I no longer felt pregnant.

It was the first time my husband was not with me during a visit. Luckily, my mom was visiting from Spain. Lennox, my mom and I were in the room when my doctor came to see me. When she asked, "How are you feeling?", I told her that I was feeling much better. "The nausea has disappeared during the last two weeks." My mention of the timing was on purpose, because I wanted to see her reaction. Immediately, I saw a sign of concern on her face. She clearly thought just what my gut was telling me. The sudden change was not normal.

My doctor told me that we were going to do an ultrasound, even though it was not due. "We'll do it just for fun," she said. But I still saw the concern on her face. Minutes later, the machine was in the room and my belly exposed and ready to check on the baby. She placed the doppler on my stomach. I could not yet see the screen. She took a deep breath and said: "I cannot see anything. The baby is gone." She proceeded to show me the screen – which I wish I had never looked at – and there it was: my completely empty uterus. I gasped "I knew it!" and quickly covered my face so my son could not see the tears flowing down.

Abruptly, I asked my mom to take my son out of the room. My poor mom was so confused. The conversation had happened in English, so she had no idea why I was crying. She looked at the doctor (who also speaks Spanish) and asked her what was going on. The doctor replied: "El bebe dejo de crecer." (The baby stopped growing). Sobbing, I again asked my mom to take my son out of the room.

I kept repeating, "I knew it. I knew it was not normal to suddenly feel better. I cannot do this anymore. I am done trying." That was when the doctor, now crying herself, confessed to me that her heart stopped when I told her how I was feeling. Once I calmed down, we started discussing options. I could take a pill to try to pass all the tissue or get a D&C. The possibility of taking the pill and not being done with the process was not something I even wanted to consider, so I chose to have a D&C.

Composing myself, I put on my sunglasses and left the room with a folder to take to the front desk to schedule my D&C. Coming out of the room, Lennox screamed from the end of the hallway, "MAMA!" I turned and gave him a big smile. My heart was broken but my little boy did not need to know that.

Placing the folder on the counter and looking down, I could not say a word. It was taking every ounce of energy to fight back tears. One of the women who worked there had become a beloved person for our family. She looked at me and said: "Remember how blessed you are to have him. I was never able to have children. You have him and he is perfect." I knew she meant well, but I was not ready to hear those words.

I do not know that you are ever ready to hear them, in all honesty. Of course, I knew I had been blessed with my beautiful son. But my heart was still hurting for the baby I had just lost and for the fact that I had to walk out of that office with the remains of the pregnancy still inside my body.

There were three days between that day and my D&C, and they were absolute torture. My mind could not stop thinking about the almost three weeks that I had walked around thinking that I was pregnant. In reality, my baby had stopped growing only days after I last saw his little heart in an ultrasound. Those thoughts haunted me day and night. As well as the thought of still having pregnancy tissue inside of my body.

The day of the D&C was an absolute blur. My husband and I went to the hospital very early in the morning. We were in a waiting room for a few minutes while my husband filled out paperwork. It felt like an out-of-body experience. Sitting there, just three days after learning I had lost another baby, and getting ready to remove the little bit that was left of another unsuccessful pregnancy.

My doctor came to see me before I was taken to the OR. I could tell she was devastated for me. This was our third miscarriage together. She had so much faith that I would get to have another baby. But, so far, it was not happening and neither of us knew why.

Once I was in the OR and sedated, she grabbed my hand, looked at me and said: "Next time I see you in an OR will be to deliver your baby." I held back tears as I began to fall asleep.

When I woke up in recovery, I started crying uncontrollably. It was over. Now it was truly over. I was not pregnant anymore. Nothing was left inside of me. It hit me so hard once I opened my eyes. A male nurse asked me: "Why are you crying?" I was in disbelief. I just managed to whisper: "Do you know why I am here? Please, bring my husband."

BARBARA'S STORY

I was 28 years old, married for two years and I got pregnant the first month after I got off my birth control pills. It was my dream come true. My husband and I went to our first OBGYN visit and I remember the nurse practitioner telling us that one in every four pregnancies ends in a loss. The thought that it could happen to me never crossed my mind. That's something that happened to other people. We were so excited to celebrate the upcoming holidays and share the good news. Thanksgiving dinner was when we told our family. There was not a dry eye in the room. This baby was so loved already.

On Dec 17th 2008, I noticed I was spotting. Immediately my heart began racing. I called my doctor and he told me to go in. They couldn't find my baby's heartbeat, so they sent me to another location to get a sonogram. Although we were able to see the baby's shape clearly, it was no longer a healthy pregnancy. The fetus had died in my womb nearly two weeks earlier. They called it a 'missed abortion.'

Those words marked me forever. I felt guilt because I kept wondering if I had done something wrong to cause this. All I could do was cry. Needless to say, that was the saddest Christmas I had experienced to date. We didn't want to partake in any celebration, we were mourning the loss of our baby. Our immediate family was as heartbroken as us, but there were others that just patted me on my shoulder and said it was never a baby to begin with. How dare they? This was my baby, and my heart told me it was a girl. Her name was Emma Nicole.

My husband bought me a puppy to help us cope with the loss and yes, it did keep our minds busy, but the wound remained. A year later God blessed us with a healthy baby boy, Rocco. And three years after that, we had Brianna Nicole. Her middle name is in honor of her angel sister.

CHAPTER 18

I AM GRIEVING WITH YOU

August 18, 2018

After dozens of messages from women giving me (unsolicited) advice as to what I should do next – what I should get tested for or whether I should even try to get pregnant again – it was a man, my brother-in-law, who sent the absolute perfect message: "I am grieving with you."

It is simply impossible to explain the dynamics of dealing with RPL (recurrent pregnancy loss), but I have learned this: the best thing you can give someone dealing with it is your compassion. This experience is a very hard roller coaster and judgment should not be part of the equation.

So, next time you want to tell a woman dealing with miscarriage what she should do next, remember my brother-in-law's words and just join the person in their pain. Their path is for them to figure out. Just extend your hand so they don't walk it alone.

> *"You are amazing girl I love your message. Thank u for being so brave and vulnerable to share this. You are truly inspiring no matter what u decide to do, I'm sending positive vibes your way."*

How ironic. The first man that I saw after the D&C that removed the remains of my latest loss was absolutely clueless as to how to react to my tears and devastation. That male nurse will never know how deeply his words affected me. How lonely and misunderstood he made me feel by dismissing my feelings only minutes after one of the most traumatic surgical procedures a woman can go through.

Yet, a man was the first person to say the perfect words to me as I mourned, for the fourth time, the loss of my unborn child. No, I did not want to hear again that God's timing was perfect. No, I did not want to hear again that everything happens for a reason. I was absolutely sick of other women telling me about what I should get tested for. I wanted and needed someone to simply hear my pain. To respect it and treat it with dignity. I needed someone to once and for all treat my loss as what it was: a loss.

My brother-in-law's words were a beacon that I held on to tightly. It was a lifeline as the days went by and, unfortunately, as I kept hearing the typical statements I did not want to hear. The intentions were good behind those words. But the dialogue really needed to change. It was a growing realization to me that one of the biggest issues with miscarriage is that the people around those who suffer such a loss rarely know how to treat them.

It is my hope that this book is not only read by women who have suffered a miscarriage, but also by loved ones who need to offer their support and may also feel lost. Remember my brother-in-law's words: "I am grieving with you." Miscarriage submerges the woman who had the loss into a very difficult grieving process. Hold her hand and walk the path with her. Offer your support without judgment, but save the advice for a later time. Maybe the time is a few months after the loss. Maybe it is never. She may never be ready to hear that she miscarried for a reason. And the reality is, more often than not, there simply is not a reason.

Four miscarriages later, I had still not been able to make sense of this path I was walking. But, if I could make an impact on how the conversation around miscarriage is handled, the pain I endured on my journey would be worth it.

There is a lot of work to do before others can understand what a woman experiences after a miscarriage. Everyone celebrates the news of a new pregnancy with such excitement. It is an amazing and powerful experience and a blessing to the woman who receives the news. Why can we not understand that when this beautiful gift is suddenly ripped from her, the pain is going to be equally as powerful?

Miscarriage seems to be the one loss that can only be understood, innately, if you have gone through it. We all seem to be capable of understanding the loss of a parent, even by those who have not experienced it. When you lose a parent, people who have not lost theirs will still understand how devastating it is. Even if we cannot relate to the loss, people will know that you will need time to mourn. Probably because we all fear the day that we see a loved one depart from our life.

Somehow we do not have the same ability to relate to the pain of a woman who has lost her baby. That needs to change. We need to consciously work to change the dialogue around miscarriage and begin to see that it also warrants the time for the woman who faces it to mourn, cope, and recover. This lack of social understanding perpetuates many women's desire to remain silent after a miscarriage instead of relying on their support system to get them through this very traumatic experience.

After one of my losses, one of my specialists and I had a conversation about this. She confessed that she had witnessed such silence among her group of close friends. As each of their OBGYN, she was the only one who knew about each of her friends' miscarriages. None of these women knew about the losses faced by the others. Out of the seven women in that group, four had suffered a miscarriage. And she was the only one who knew.

Hearing her say that broke my heart. Someone who has not suffered a miscarriage probably cannot imagine that the stigma that accompanies that loss is so severe, that you may choose to not even share it with your close girlfriends. Imagine the loneliness that follows when you allow yourself to go to that level of isolation. And all because you have learned through watching others that the social support is not quite there.

We need to change that. One conversation at a time. I urge you to be the person on the other side who simply listens and offers unconditional support. Cry with her, hold her, tell her you feel her pain, that you understand and that she is not alone. Do not overthink your words. Simplicity is key. Just listen to what your heart would need to hear if you were her. Sometimes, it may take just five words: "I am grieving with you."

CATHERINE'S STORY

I have been there three times and it was devastating. I couldn't function for so long. You are beautiful inside and out. I would like to say to other women experiencing the same, "I am here for you." We never know the why. We only know we have to trust and have faith. I made it through and I didn't have the strength and courage you do. You're a blessing to me.

―――――――

Join the movement. Share these stories so that we all have a voice. #TheLightAfterLoss

- @siramara
- Sandy Bodeau
- @sanbodeau

CHAPTER 19

THE ELEPHANT IN THE ROOM

August 22, 2018

Had my first big meeting yesterday after taking a few days off, and everybody froze when I went in the room. I thought: "my dress must be really cute." Then I realized what was happening. No one knew what to do.

Their reaction made me think about what is the "right" thing to do. I knew almost any approach would make me cry but I definitely did not want silence.

I'm truly hoping to help end the stigma around miscarriage. I know it must be uncomfortable and sad to approach somebody going through such a dark time, but remember that love and compassion are always well received.

When you see somebody after losing a loved one, you tell them you are sorry. When you see somebody after surgery, you tell them you are happy that they are recovering nicely. This is no different. It is about pain and it is about healing. It is about love and it is about loss.

If silence was not an option, what would YOU have done if you were in that room? Let's find a better way to address women dealing with this heartbreaking situation.

#ihadamiscarriage

"Beautiful message and so true. We need to share what we would want to hear."

Eight days had passed since my fourth miscarriage and I was still bleeding from the D&C. My heart, obviously, was bleeding even harder. Over the last few days, I had spent every second that I could find crying in my room. Thankfully, my mom was there and took charge of taking care of Lennox and the house. My heart and soul were broken, matching my body that had once again failed me. Every step I took was labored as I walked around the house staring at walls, doors, and furniture. Surrounded by a foggy haze, I was simply lost.

While trying to be respectful of my feelings and allowing myself to go through my healing process, I also needed air. The pain I felt was suffocating and staying home in hiding was not helping that. When dealing with loss there is a difficult balance that needs to be found between allowing your feelings to be fully felt and not allowing them to drag you into a darkness that you struggle to get out of. When I decided to go to my first post-miscarriage meeting, it was that balance I was trying to find.

Clothes shape how you feel; something I always taught my clients as a fashion stylist. So the clothes I wore needed to remind me of who I was, even though I was not feeling like that person at the moment. The dress I chose had a star pattern. (Superstar is the nickname that my Madrid friends gave me when I moved to the U.S.) That dress was matched with a pair of red pumps. Red had been the color I used a lot when I worked for the U.S. Senate. Women in politics are not really known for their daring or colorful outfits, so I was often discouraged from wearing red. But it was because of this preconceived idea that I always chose red for big meetings during my political career. The point was quickly made to all in the room that I was confident in who I was and no one was going to make me someone that I was not. So, red pumps it was, and high ones at that.

This was a meeting with a local PR company that offered me a fantastic opportunity to partner with the City of Coral Gables. That is the Miami neighborhood where I live. The pitch was to showcase the many great amenities that visitors could enjoy during a visit. We love where we live, so, in spite of how broken I was inside, I thought I would be able to have a successful meeting.

Walking into the room, it was instantly clear that everyone knew about my miscarriage. The announcement had come just a few days earlier but, somehow, it shocked me to see their faces. They all looked at me as if a ghost had just entered the room. The loud laughter and chatter I had heard as I approached the room had disappeared instantly.

Only a few seconds, but it felt like an eternity. I froze by the door and everyone just froze with me. No one moved. No one talked. No one did anything for those excruciating few seconds. No red pumps or star patterns could give me strength to face that situation. All I wanted to do was to turn around and run away crying.

Finally, the president of the company got up from her chair and came towards me. We had been speaking via email for a few weeks now. She re-introduced herself and invited me to find a seat. My body was literally shaking as I walked in. Lots of awkward introductions followed. No one looked me in the eye, even when speaking to me directly. The entire meeting was spent fighting back tears. My voice shook each time anyone asked me a question.

The presentation about my approach to present the campaign on social media was an absolute disaster. I could not remember half of the things I wanted to say. The very few I could remember were presented in an unfavorable way. Their eyes felt like swords thrown at me each time they met with mine.

In hindsight, I wish I had stopped right there and said: "Excuse me if I do not sound very prepared for the meeting. I was pregnant just a few days ago. But I just had a miscarriage and I am really struggling. I am doing my best to push through and do life, but you may need to bear with me as I figure out a way to do so." But I did not. Instead, I became part of the silence. The silence I dreaded myself so much and found so cruel during the miscarriage mourning process.

Leaving the meeting, I was absolutely defeated. It was clear that I was not going to get the campaign. (I did not). But that was not why I felt defeated. I felt defeated because I had not been able to speak up about what was going on in that room. After four miscarriages, I needed to be heard. But I could not expect others to hear words that I was not saying myself.

Once I got home, I thought about how I could have handled things differently. Expecting others to know what we want to hear after a miscarriage is not fair. We need to express our feelings so we guide those outside of the situation. We all need episodes like the one I went through during that PR meeting to become less and less common. I did not know how, but I was determined to do my part to figure out how to change the conversation around miscarriage.

JULIANNA'S STORY

I had a miscarriage and an ectopic pregnancy within three months. It sent me into a deep depression. I only saw two options: suicide or chasing my teenage dream of becoming a psychologist. Fortunately, I chose the latter. I wrote my thesis on the resignification of femininity in fertile women.

Today, I help many women to find courage within themselves through elements other than maternity to define their feminity. I am so grateful for the exposure that you are giving to this topic. Society has made it an invisible topic worldwide. I am sure that your words are a source of support for many women like me during these trials.

Join the movement. Share these stories so that we all have a voice. #TheLightAfterLoss

@siramara

Sandy Bodeau

@sanbodeau

CHAPTER 20

FIND THE INSPIRATION

August 25, 2018

My biggest takeaway from my day with the @instagram team yesterday: "FIND THE INSPIRATION IN INSTAGRAM."

It has taken me six years of using this app to fully understand this. From my initial focus in entrepreneurship to then focusing on fashion to then focusing on lifestyle, it has been through my struggle with RPL (recurrent pregnancy loss) that I found my ultimate inspiration in Instagram: YOU.

You, when you told me that my honesty has helped you through your healing process

You, when you told me that you finally asked for help to cope with your loss after I shared my journey

You, when you told me that you were ready to give up but now feel empowered to try to get pregnant again because I've shared that I will not give up

YOU with the hundreds of messages that you've shared with me during this journey that I never expected to be my own have inspired me to turn my suffering into a purpose and to see #thelightafterloss

> *"I love this!! I adore that mindset with this crazy Insta world. And I love that it connects to people all over who can inspire us!"*

That was the day that I wanted to avoid at all costs. It was the meeting that I wrote about in the first chapter and it became a day that I will never forget. It is the day I realized that I needed to write this book.

Excitedly, I had accepted an invitation to attend a meeting at the Facebook offices in Miami. But that was prior to my fourth miscarriage. After the miscarriage, and its very public announcement, the last place I wanted to be was surrounded by a bunch of people who knew that I had lost another baby.

My husband helped me realize it was an opportunity that I would be disappointed to have missed. So, I agreed to go and make the most out of the day. Little did I know that the encounter with my friend Jeannette, who treated me with kindness and humanity, would be the starting point in my effort to expand my voice beyond Instagram. It was the simplest of gestures. One that you would think would come so naturally to many people. And yet, this was the first time that someone had treated me correctly over the course of four miscarriages. A hug. A smile. Just three words – "How are you?" The simple acknowledgement that I was probably not okay.

Jeannette's actions not only showed me the path that I wanted to take from that point forward when it came to speaking publicly about my miscarriages. Her compassion also helped me focus during the meeting and truly absorb the message that Instagram had prepared for us. Every person in the room was not only invited to attend as an influencer, but also as a parent. Instagram was introducing a guide for parents to help their children navigate the platform in a safe and enjoyable manner.

As part of the presentation, we learned about hashtags that had become a movement way beyond the platform. The #kindcomments hashtag was created by Instagram, and the company started an initiative that turned walls in cities around the world into colorful murals inspiring #KindComments. Instagram encouraged people to visit one of the walls, take a photo or video and share a #KindComment to make someone's day.

As I type this, the hashtag has been shared on 364,000 posts. All those people were able to positively impact others after having found the inspiration on Instagram. We'll never know how many people have been able to be reached by those messages, but I would guess that millions of eyes have witnessed the powerful movement.

What was clear to me was that I could also create that kind of impact. The confirmation of the impact came from women all over the world. Women who messaged me every single time I spoke about my miscarriages. Women who let me know how understood they felt after reading my posts. Women who needed to know that they were not alone.

Many of the comments included the phrase: "you are so inspiring." In reality, they were the ones that inspired my newfound purpose. The isolation, the shame, and the guilt – none of those things were fair. After months spent privately sharing with each of the women that reached out, I was driven to take a public stance. It was time to use the inspiration that I had found in Instagram. Hopefully, I could impact many others through sharing my difficult journey. After years of using the platform as a marketing tool, I realized that Instagram had led me to find my inspiration.

After all the horrible loss I had gone through in less than three years, I had found a light. The light was the power of connection and community that came from having shared my experience of pregnancy loss and the impact it had on others. This light became my guide to show me the direction I needed to go with my miscarriage journey.

KIM'S STORY

I have been there. In my second pregnancy, my doctor figured out I was about 18 weeks pregnant based on the measurements but he could not find a heartbeat. I had an ultrasound later that day that confirmed that my baby was gone. My body just had not figured it out yet. Thankfully, my doctor scheduled my D&C for the morning. Even though that happened 19 years ago, I still remember the feeling of loss. I am grateful that women today have these kinds of spaces to speak about this topic and that you have so bravely decided to share your experiences to help others.

———

Join the movement. Share these stories so that we all have a voice. #TheLightAfterLoss

@siramara

Sandy Bodeau

@sanbodeau

CHAPTER 21

THE FIRST STEP

August 28, 2018

THE FIRST STEP IS ALWAYS THE HARDEST.

Remember that when you try to overcome a fear. That is me now trying to overcome the fear of facing friends/coworkers after my miscarriage.

The truth is that you never really feel prepared to face a fear. You either choose to conquer it or let it conquer you and your life. I want to encourage you all to choose to always be the CONQUEROR.

We can do this. #TheLightAfterLoss

"You are just incredible! I'm sure you have helped and empowered so many women and made them feel comfortable to at least talk about it."

Talk about it. Yes, that was my first step towards turning my pain into my purpose. To this day, I have not found a magical formula to heal myself from my recurrent pregnancy loss, but I have definitely learned that simply talking about it helps tremendously. So, I decided to talk. And I decided to do so in the most natural way.

To begin with, I decided to admit that I was struggling. It was time to talk about those first few encounters and how difficult they are. If my mission was to teach others to approach women who have had a miscarriage naturally, I needed to lead by example. Normalization of this topic was much needed.

While there is a lot of pain associated with miscarriage, there is also a lot of potential for growth. I was learning that about myself. It was a subject that I would have preferred not to be an expert on, but the numbers told a different story. Only 1% of women suffer three or more miscarriages. That placed me solidly within a small group of women who were subject matter experts.

There were two things that I could do about that. I could feel sorry for myself or I could use my extended experience to guide others through their own mourning process. It had become clear to me that other women were connecting with me through social media on the subject to feel empowered. If I could encourage myself to face my fear after four miscarriages, it felt like compelling evidence that they could too.

The first step is hard. And it is okay to fear those first few encounters after miscarriage. They are not easy, and not only because you feel observed and pitied. What is often most difficult to comprehend is how quickly the world has moved on while time has frozen for you. You are still trying to pick your heart's pieces from the ground. But all the while, meetings keep happening, birthdays keep being celebrated, and life in general has not stopped for one second.

That is why the first step is not only the hardest but also the most important. You decide where you want it to take you. There is no rush. Let the world keep moving at its hectic pace. You should take the time to regroup and step back on only when you are ready. Your first step is going to take you into a new direction. It is essential that you choose wisely where you step. Light is on one side. Darkness on the other. The direction may not be obvious from the start, so step with care. Remember, this is a journey.

The process will vary by the person, but be sure to make your decisions from a place of light. Whether that decision means trying to have another baby right away, waiting for two years to try again, deciding that trying to conceive is not something you can do anymore…it can be done from a place of light or from a place of darkness. With hindsight, I am sure that you will feel better about your decision if you make it from a place of light.

That was definitely my case. Two weeks after having my D&C, I was not in the mindset to even think about exactly when we would try again. But I knew that we would be back to trying to have our second baby sooner rather than later. And I knew that because I was making that decision from a place of light. It was not time to give up or change paths. And I knew that my newfound purpose would help me find the strength to face anything else life may have in store for me.

The messages kept coming. They never stopped shocking me. Untold stories of women who had silently suffered for years. Isolated. Many of them writing from a place of absolute darkness. Choosing to break their silence because a stranger on the internet was showing them that it was okay to talk about it. Not only that it was okay but that there was lots of power in those that were willing to share their stories.

Using my own journey, I was able to show others how they could have the same exact impact in people's lives and, little by little, the messages began becoming public. The stories that were mostly shared via private message started to show up in the comments on my posts. And I could tell that others were reading them. Many of them were unable to reply back. But the likes on those comments told me that other women were finding company in the middle of their isolation.

My first step towards a place of light was making others take action. It was humbling to be in that position. Opening up the conversation about miscarriage on my Instagram account was creating a chain reaction between other women who were facing my same challenges. It was impossible to know whether or not I would succeed at having another child. But I started to believe that there was already a lot of success in my journey. I was becoming its conqueror.

SUSAN'S STORY

I have had three miscarriages and one of them ended up with a D&C, like yours. We had fires during that time, and people were evacuating. All I knew was that I still had a baby inside of me. It was a feeling that I will never forget. Thanks for opening up and sharing your story with others. I wish I had a chance to read more about it when I was going through my losses. Bless you and your family.

––––––––––

Join the movement. Share these stories so that we all have a voice. #TheLightAfterLoss

@siramara
Sandy Bodeau
@sanbodeau

CHAPTER 22

THE ANNIVERSARY PARTY

September 5, 2018

It has been almost a month since my last miscarriage, and I must confess that even though you see me on Instagram, I have been kind of hiding. From my friends, from public events and from TV.

A little over a year ago, my dear @patriciaproducer called me to ask me if I wanted to be part of a little show that was about to start. That little show is now #1 in ratings and today it was its first year anniversary.

When Patricia called me to ask me to come back for the celebration show, I truly wanted to say no. But I actually wanted to be there to celebrate with all the people who have worked so very hard to make this show a success.

I was afraid to go through the doors. I was afraid that I was going to break down (and ruin the STUNNING makeup by @pelusamakeup). Instead, I just felt so much love! Everybody welcomed me with open arms and I was so glad to be there with my TV family.

Now, I am ready to reunite with you, our dear viewers and I have an AMAZING segment ready for you at 1 pm. #thelightafterloss

"My Sandy, you are a warrior. I admire your bravery so much, and I am so happy that you had the courage to come to the show today. And your segment rocked, per usual! We love you, and this is your home!" – Patricia

My producer, Patricia, wrote that comment. We had spoken a few days prior about joining the team for the anniversary party. She knew what I was going through, but I am very glad that she pushed me to join. I was not in the mood for parties, but this show was very special to me. It was a show that had grown so much in spite of having started so small. And I had been part of it since day one. Facing people was unappealing, but I knew that it was going to be a celebration that I would be honored to be a part of.

Just by attending, I knew that it would send a strong message to those suffering from their own losses. Yes, I was sad and confused. But I was also ready to show other women that I could face my biggest fears and come out of hiding. Because of my good fortune to have a platform where people visited to be impacted by my words, it was also important to show them with actions what I was made of.

My friend Luis Aponte often dresses me for my TV segments and events. In addition to being a star fashion designer, he was also a good friend who knew the pain I was suffering. My request was a statement outfit. This was not just my return to the show. It was a coming out party to let the world know I was back! They would see that, although I was hurting, I was not broken.

It was also a conscious decision to call my forever makeup artist, my dear Pelusa (may she rest in peace) to do my makeup. Pelusa had been there when I started TV as a bright eyed novice. And she had a knack for always making me feel and look like a queen. This was one of the times that I knew I needed Pelusa and her magic touch. She did not disappoint.

At 5 am in the morning, I drove myself to the Univision studios to make my TV comeback. It was just a few weeks after my fourth miscarriage. Sparkly pants, lace top and the most fabulous makeup a girl could dream of. While still fearful of those first few encounters, I was ready.

Always among the very first to arrive at the studio, this day was no different and I had a chance to be alone and catch my breath. A few minutes after my arrival, my friend and host of the show, Alberto Sardiñas, saw me backstage. He immediately came towards me, gave me a big hug, smiled at me and said, "We are so happy that you are here." I smiled back, thanked him and showed him that I was going to be okay. Encounters like the one with Alberto kept happening. It was clear that having openly spoken about the ups and downs of the last few days had helped make those encounters less awkward. People were beginning to see that if I could treat my loss naturally, so could they.

But, it did happen again. Minutes before the show went live, a man approached me and said "Hi." No hug – as he usually did – no eye contact. We made small talk. In the middle of it, he said, "Yeah, you were not here that day. It was when that happened to you." He was still not looking at me in the eye.

Obviously, I knew what he meant. But this was an opportunity for growth for both of us. Breaking down publicly was still a real fear. But it was a fear I would face. And I would help him overcome the fear of saying anything wrong after a loss. "When? Oh, do you mean when I had my miscarriage?" He immediately looked at me. For the first time in the minutes he had been talking to me, he made eye contact. By speaking directly about 'that' thing that had happened to me, I was no longer invisible to him. It was a step in the right direction for us both.

No longer would I be invisible. That stopped being something I wanted to be on that very day. Invisibility was not what I deserved. I deserved compassion. And compassion is also what you deserve if you have suffered a miscarriage.

The need to hide is completely understandable. And sometimes it is necessary. But I also want to encourage you to take those little steps towards not allowing yourself to be invisible to the world. The world cannot help us if we hide. It is up to us to show them that we are here. That we are surviving a terribly tragic loss. That we are hurting. The isolation that comes from invisibility is not what we need. We need to be seen so that we can receive the love, compassion, and understanding that we deserve.

CHRISTINA'S STORY

I have had two miscarriages and I have struggled with infertility for years after them. We have tried everything. It has been really hard. At the same time, posts like yours let me know that I am not alone and that, if it is meant to be, it will happen.

I admire your strength in sharing with us on Instagram. I am a super private person, but I am always so grateful for those who do share, because it is a needed reminder that so many people go through it. I am so lucky to have an amazing marriage and support system. Most of my girlfriends have two or three kids already, which makes me happy for them but it is also tough. It is just crazy that some people can get pregnant with one try, some after years of trying, and some never. You are never taught that when you are growing up, you know?

———————

Join the movement. Share these stories so that we all have a voice. #TheLightAfterLoss

🄾 @siramara

🄵 Sandy Bodeau

🄳 @sanbodeau

CHAPTER 23

THE FESTIVAL

September 15, 2018

From my speech tonight at the @savingsicklecelllives festival:

"I must confess that I did not want to show up today. I committed to being here two months ago. I was pregnant then. Unfortunately, I lost that baby a month ago, and when you lose a baby you don't really feel like going to a music festival. But I stand on this stage tonight holding my son, because I want him to learn that when you get the privilege of helping others, you show up. When it is important, you show up. When you can make an impact, you show up. And when it saves lives, YOU SHOW UP."

Thank you, dear Naomi for giving me the privilege of being part of this. #thelightafterloss

"Sometimes showing up isn't easy at all. Proud of you."

Before I had my fourth miscarriage, I had been looking forward to attending the Saving Sickle Cell Lives festival. When I was just 11 months old, I was diagnosed with sickle cell disease. That diagnosis was a big part of my life during my childhood. While I had reached a point as an adult when the disorder no longer ruled my life, I was honored that the Saving Sickle Cell Lives organization had contacted me to get involved and advocate with them.

Coincidentally, one of the doctors who ran the organization, Dr. Thomas Harris, had been my hematologist during Lennox's pregnancy.

He was a kind man and a special kind of doctor. Knowing that he was part of the organization made me even more excited to help.

But that was before the miscarriage. Now, as the day of the festival came along, the idea of being around crowds was not something I felt ready for. Still, I decided to keep my commitment to them because I would have later regretted not having shown up for a cause so near and dear to my heart.

Like I had in the past for the album release party, I talked myself into thinking that being in a crowded space could actually be good. The hectic pace, the music and the many people around me would protect me from feeling too exposed. There was also safety knowing that no one except the organizer, Naomi, knew about my miscarriage. So I would not feel like I was walking with a target on my back, as it had often felt during the last few weeks.

The first person we saw when we got to the event was Dr. Harris. He was so happy to see us and he beamed with the infectious energy that he has. It was the first time we had seen each other since my pregnancy with Lennox. It was so nice to introduce him to the baby that was in my belly when we met. We chatted with him for a little bit and then went to find Naomi.

Naomi was running all over the place, as is typical for a good festival manager. She was doing everything she could to make everything run smoothly. We met her husband and two of her beautiful children. Looking around, I told myself that I was proud to have made it to the event. It was good to be there. It was good to be helpful.

But then, Naomi came to ask me to give a speech. That changed my mood immediately. Being there mixed with the crowds and having small talk conversations with people was one thing. Getting on a stage was a completely different story.

Every negative emotion swirled around within me and I told my husband that I was not going to do it. There was no way I could go on that stage and have all eyes on me. Everyone would know that I'd had a miscarriage just by looking at me, or at least that was how I felt. The target was back and their eyes would be shooting straight into my heart.

My husband always knows when to push me, because he knows how I will feel afterwards if I decide not to do something. He encouraged me to consider doing a little speech. A small part of me began to believe that he was probably right and that I could do it. But it was when I looked at my beautiful baby boy that I realized that not only could I do it, but that I had to do it. This was an important battle in the fight against invisibility. And I was going to lead by example. It was time to show my little boy that even during times of adversity, you have to show up when it matters.

Waiting for my turn backstage, my heart was racing. Giving a speech was not on my radar, so I had nothing prepared. And I was always prepared for these sorts of things. My legs were shaking. My hands were sweating. So I called my husband and asked him to bring my son. Once Lennox was in my arms, I knew exactly what I was going to say. We were going to go on stage together.

There are a lot of memories that stand out from that speech. There were the confused looks as I began with the line "I did not want to be here today." But it certainly got everyone's attention. There was a shocked and sad look on Dr. Harris's face when I shared that I had just had a miscarriage as he was standing just offstage after having given his speech. It was a compassionate look that told me "I am grieving with you."

But what I remember the most were the faces looking at me when I had finished my speech. They were faces of gratitude. These were the faces of moms whose kids were there because the organization provided much-needed help. They were thankful that I had decided that their kids were important; that they deserved to be seen. By choosing to fight my own desire to remain invisible, I had helped give others visibility. And my son was my witness.

It is important to put yourself out there sometimes. You never know when something you might have dreaded being a part of turns out to be one of the proudest moments of your life.

NORA'S STORY

It was my first pregnancy. I did not even know that I was pregnant. I thought that I was having a heavier than normal period. I decided to go to the doctor when the bleeding got intense. They sent me to the hospital immediately and I learned there that I was having a miscarriage. I needed a D&C.

Even though I never got to even be excited about being pregnant, it still hurt terribly. I felt like a part of me was gone. I have never told this story to anybody. Not even my family. My husband is the only one who knows and now you. I need to tell you as a way to free myself from carrying the burden of keeping the secret for so long. Thank you for giving me the chance to do so.

———————

Join the movement. Share these stories so that we all have a voice. #TheLightAfterLoss

⬚ @siramara
⬚ Sandy Bodeau
⬚ @sanbodeau

CHAPTER 24

FACES OF FERTILITY

October 15, 2018

ALWAYS remember that we're all on a journey called 'life' and things are not always as they seem.

After sharing the news of #MeghanMarkle's pregnancy on my stories, I got a DM that said: "I hate women who get pregnant so easily."

Me: "I am one of those women you hate. I have been pregnant five times in three years. You may have noticed that I only have one child. I hope that you can turn that hatred into hope and that you get the baby you so badly wish."

I am proud to join the #FacesOfFertility campaign to help create the much needed conversation about pregnancy and infant loss. Please share your story using the #FacesOfFertility hashtag

"What a beautiful caption. I wish I could hug you."

Being chosen to be part of the Faces of Fertility campaign was a big honor for me. But it was more than that. It was an indicator that my voice, the voice I found through sharing my journey, was being heard. My vulnerable posts that were initially shared as a way to open up about my heartache were impacting others. But that direct message about Meghan Markle showed me that there was still a lot of work to be done. And I was ready to do my part.

When I read the words "I hate women who get pregnant so easily" I cried. It felt like a big slap in the face, because I was one of 'them.' I had always become pregnant very easily. And yet, my body was not as 'perfect' as this woman seemed to believe. Her words made me feel like I belonged to an elite group, but I was part of a lesser category. The one with a defect.

Yes, I was able to get pregnant easily. But, no, my body was not able to carry those 'easy' pregnancies to term. The comment had really stirred up my insecurities. And now I learned that some women felt hatred towards those who do not struggle to get pregnant.

Hatred is a cruel reaction. But I knew that this person was not cruel. The infertility journey had simply created some very negative feelings within her. And it was likely that many other women out there could be feeling the same way.

So, I decided to speak up. For the ones getting pregnant easily and able to carry pregnancies to term. For the ones like me, getting pregnant easily but unable to carry all pregnancies to term. And for the ones suffering due to their inability to get pregnant and being so hurt that they had turned their pain into hatred towards others. This division was unfair for everyone and, again, I chose not to stay silent. We needed to band together, not tear each other apart.

Those strong feelings of hatred made me reflect on my own feelings. While I had not experienced hatred towards anyone with an easier path than mine, I often struggled watching some of my friends bringing their babies into the world. Particularly ones who did so at the time when one of my angel babies would have been born. I had even stopped looking at the pictures of those babies and quickly scrolled past them to avoid the stabbing heartache I felt knowing that the baby I lost would be that age. In my own way, I admitted, I was participating in the division of 'us' versus 'them.' 'Us.' the ones suffering silently. 'Them,' the lucky ones who had an easy path.

That was going to change today. I was going to do better and be better. It was time to change the narrative. I was one of 'Us.' 'Us' being every single woman who chooses to be a mother, regardless of the outcome of that choice. That was the only group I was going to be part of. No more avoiding looking at other babies. No more comparing my journey with anyone else's. And no more allowing people to believe that feeling hatred towards others with a different path was healthy in any shape or form.

Unity. That is what we need through this journey. Not division, nor hatred, nor avoidance. A united front of women who have a common wish to get one of life's biggest privileges: that of creating a life. It is a powerful bond that we share. The focus is not on what any of us ends up obtaining at the end of the journey. The focus is the journey itself.

Deciding to start a family requires an incredible amount of faith and hope. Making that decision immediately puts us in a very vulnerable position. For as much as we may want to create life, we do not get the ultimate say on whether or not we will get our wish. So, let us all remember to be compassionate towards each other. Some will conquer the journey more easily while others may struggle through it. We all share a common goal, regardless of our journey.

TAMARA'S STORY

I have had four miscarriages. The first one was at eight months of pregnancy. I cried day and night. It took us a year and a half to be able to try again. I lost my second pregnancy at 10 weeks. Even though doctors explained to me that a miscarriage means that the baby was not genetically healthy, I started feeling bad about myself. I did not know of anybody who had suffered two miscarriages. I was convinced that we were sick and that was what was creating the miscarriages.

We went through extensive testing and no abnormality was found in either of us. With the information and filled with hope, we tried again. I got pregnant really fast, again, and again I lost that third baby at eight weeks of pregnancy. It took us two years to try again. I lost that fourth baby at seven weeks of pregnancy.

I never had any problem getting pregnant. But these recurrent losses created a very uncomfortable environment for me, on top of my own heartache. My friends and family started to talk behind my back. They pitied me. They wondered what was wrong with me. But no one came to me and asked: "How are you doing?" I went into a deep depression. I started having panic attacks. My doctor encouraged me to start seeing a psychologist and it helped me tremendously.

It was during treatment that I found you on Instagram. After reading about your recurrent pregnancy losses, I finally did not feel alone and lost in this world. I finally learned that I was not the only woman going through this. I also learned from you that I should not give up. I am currently 18 weeks pregnant and everything is going great.

CHAPTER 25

THANKFUL FOR HARDSHIP

November 24, 2018

The stomach flu kept me from doing my #Thanksgiving post but it is my favorite holiday and it is a week-long celebration in my book, so here I am.

I thought long and hard about what I was most thankful for this year. It made me realize that it is easy to be thankful for the good things in our lives. But what about the not so good? Don't they matter? Don't they change us in a way that can, indeed, be good?

This year, I am thankful for all the hardship I endured. While I am definitely not thankful to have lost two babies, I am thankful for the person that came out of those experiences.

Hardship that showed me that my family will forever rally around me in times of need.

Hardship that taught me to rebuild a broken heart because, above it all, I believe in happiness.

Hardship that taught me that life is much better when we are capable of giving thanks when the road is not what we expected

Hardship that did not make me bitter, jealous, or angry but hopeful, faithful, and more humble.

"So well said!! Hardships are what bring us together and change us!"

It is very easy to be thankful when great things are happening in our lives. When we set goals and we reach them, it is natural to give thanks and feel grateful. There is even more power in being thankful for experiences that were not easy to go through. That is a lesson I had learned on my journey.

As the commenter said, my hardship had changed me. It made me stop and look at my life with a deep sense of gratitude. In all honesty, I would rather have had a much easier path. My choice would have been to have endured less heartbreak. But given that this was my path, I chose to be grateful for the hardship. And I was truly grateful for the opportunity to become a better person by way of the lessons that the hardship had taught me.

But I was most grateful for the opportunity to help others by showing a different perspective about loss and hardship. It was a blessing that I had a platform to share my experience. Rather than it simply being a personal journey, I was fortunate that my journey could be an inspiring one. And I was happy to be able to show people that even during darkness you can find reasons to be grateful. That you could even be grateful for the darkness itself.

Our journey through darkness is a great time to reflect. Why is this my path? What can I learn from it? Who do I want to become once I come out of the dark? Those are the questions that I kept asking myself.

It had been one year since I began to publicly share my struggle to carry another pregnancy to term. I was grateful for the lessons learned over that period. Along the way, I came to believe that this path allowed me to reach this level of vulnerability in order for me to connect with women all over the world. The pain and darkness that these other women and I shared provided the opportunity to form an unbreakable bond.

Another key lesson was the immense power of social media. Those little Instagram squares that we all used for fun in the beginning had become a window through which one could actually make an impact in the world. Finally, I learned exactly who I wanted to become after going through the darkness. Armed with my own expertise, and a community of fellow warriors, I wanted to be a voice of hope.

This was not the first time I had gone through hardship. But this time it was certainly different. For example, when facing financial hardship, I could work more and seek out better opportunities. I could make a plan, as I did, to further my education and create a better professional life for myself. But this was a different situation. There was nothing within my power that could be done to force Mother Nature to allow me to carry a pregnancy to term. So when it came to actually overcoming my hardship, I was entirely powerless.

For that reason, I chose gratitude and continued to focus on the growth. I could not judge my success on whether or not I reached my dream of having another baby. While I would continue to do all that I could to make that dream a reality, ultimately, it was not up to me. What was up to me was my choice of how to face the challenge. It was the choice to see it as an opportunity to grow. And it was the desire to seize this opportunity to serve those who had been listening to my new voice for over a year now.

When it comes to hardship, overcoming may not mean that you actually arrive at what you previously thought was your ideal destination. You may overcome without arriving anywhere at all. Or you may overcome by changing the path, even the entire narrative, and set a new destination. In the end, the best way to overcome may be the growth you make, the journey itself, or even the impact you make.

If you get to grow, if you get to serve, and if you get to make an impact, look at that hurdle with as much gratitude as you have in your soul. Hardship chose you and you chose to turn it into a good thing for others. That is a victory right there!

CAMILA'S STORY

I was six weeks pregnant when I found out that I was expecting a baby. I saw my doctor and he told me that everything looked fine but the baby was measuring a bit small. Two days later, I had to go to the ER due to severe vomiting. Everything still looked fine with my baby. I started bleeding a week later. Scared, I went to see my doctor again. He told me that spotting during early pregnancy was normal but noticed, again, that the baby was measuring small.

Another week went by and I started bleeding again. My doctor ordered bed rest for a few days. On my first day out of bed, the bleeding got heavier and heavier. I started cramping badly and felt my little baby come out of me when I went to use the bathroom.

I started crying hysterically and asked my husband to take me to the ER. I walked in and told the nurse that I was there because I had had a miscarriage. The doctor later confirmed that I had lost my baby. I did not need a D&C. I left the hospital only a few hours later, seemingly, the same way I had arrived. No one comforted me. No one acknowledged that I had just lost a baby. They simply sent me home.

I cried myself to sleep for days. I drank heavily for days. I felt so lost and powerless. I decided to give my baby a name as the only way I found to grieve the loss of a person I had never met. Her name was Pilar.

Join the movement. Share these stories so that we all have a voice. #TheLightAfterLoss

@siramara

Sandy Bodeau

@sanbodeau

DEAR BODY

December 12, 2018

Dear Body,

We had a rocky start. We were told you would make my life difficult due to my sickle cell anemia. That you would prevent me from having a 'normal' life and from being an active child.

But we proved them all wrong. We overcame so much. I got to live a good childhood and reached my dream to become a long distance runner against all odds. We, dear body, felt on top of the world.

Then, I had my 1st miscarriage and it hurt thinking that we were no longer a good team. Then came three more miscarriages and I simply felt betrayed by you, my lifelong partner.

It has taken me four months after my last miscarriage to realize that you do not give up on your partner. You weather storms together. You walk through the fire hand-in-hand. You pick each other up at your weakest.

Dear body, I forgive you for the things I wish you could do for me and you may not be able to, as much as I hope that you forgive me for losing faith in you. No matter what the future holds, we are in this together.

"So beautiful! I love your words. So freeing."

Freedom was exactly what I had been needing for the last few months. Freedom from the guilt I felt for being unable to give my husband the baby we both so badly wanted. Freedom from shame caused by what I felt was a defective body. Freedom from constantly thinking about ovulation calendars, pregnancy tests, and monthly disappointments. All I wanted to do was feel like myself again. That was incredibly hard because I barely recognized my body when I looked in the mirror.

From the outside, I did not look that different. I am sure no one noticed the changes. But I could see the footprint of my miscarriages all over my body. It was in my tired eyes from sleep deprivation. It was in my increasingly gray hair. It was in the bloat that I was unable to get rid of due to the crazy hormonal imbalance that three consecutive miscarriages had caused. Having a constant reminder of my losses each time I looked in the mirror had become its own nightmare. A nightmare that I so badly wanted to leave behind.

Despite those feelings, I tried to remind myself how appreciative I had always been for the things my body had done for me. Most important of all was the immense gift of my beautiful baby boy. Even still, I struggled to give my body grace because I truly wanted to have another baby, and it was not happening. No matter how much healthier I ate or how much I exercised, my body was not giving me what I hoped it would.

But the bitterness had become too much for me to carry through life. It was time for forgiveness. It was time to simply cherish what my body had done for me and stop looking at it as a broken machine. My body was not broken. It was on its own journey towards becoming a better version of itself. Just like I was trying to do mentally. Whether or not that better version would give me another child was yet to be seen. But I simply needed to trust my body again, regardless of the outcome. This was the very same powerful 'machine' that had created my son. I was going to give it my trust again.

Just a few weeks earlier, I had started collaborating on a new TV show. Professionally speaking, I felt on top of the world. But my struggle with body image after my miscarriages was haunting me. It was as if everyone could see that I looked different. "Can they tell that I have a bit of a belly?" "Are they thinking that I used to be thinner?"

I am now sure that no one could see what I could see, but that was all I could think about each time I put on my 'TV clothes.' As someone who works in fashion, I was always expected to look the part. But never had I felt more insecure wearing the beautiful outfits I got to wear.

This is yet another unspoken aspect of pregnancy loss. It is the mental impact that the physical changes have on the woman who goes through a loss. It is hard enough not to recognize yourself on the inside, after an emotional whirlwind. But carrying the scars of the failure all over my body was hard to come to grips with. That is why I decided to openly talk about it for the first time.

The beginning of my own physical healing was just starting. And it was starting from the inside. Through forgiveness and compassion. Through understanding and empathy. Just like I had done weeks before, opening up about my mental struggle, opening up about how I felt about my body was a necessary step towards freeing myself from the anger I felt towards it. A new day had come. I was freeing my body of the responsibility of giving me another baby.

ANA MARIA'S STORY

I just read your last post and I wanted to share with you that I have had five losses. Two of them with an ex-boyfriend years ago. Now, I have had three with my husband.

I am not going to give up. I will exhaust all my options. I really want to be a mother. I do not know why I cannot stay pregnant. All my losses are around seven weeks. We have not found a reason. Which makes me really angry. Why me? Why do I have to fight so hard to have what others get so easily? Why is my body not doing what it was created to do? I am getting older and the possibility of maybe not having a baby scares me to death.

Thank you for sharing your story with us. I feel less alone every time I read one of your posts. I truly hope that you also get to have the baby you are praying for.

Join the movement. Share these stories so that we all have a voice. #TheLightAfterLoss

@siramara

Sandy Bodeau

@sanbodeau

CHAPTER 27

WAITING FOR 2019

December 31, 2018

WAITING FOR YOU, 2019!

"I know it has been a year to forget for you." That message came from a friend. Initially, I did not know what she meant. But then I realized that she was talking about my two miscarriages.

Have I forgotten my pain? No. But time and time again I choose to keep the moments I want to **REMEMBER** closer to my heart.

I remember Lennox's first birthday and the many loved ones who celebrated his life with us.

I remember laughing until crying many more times than I can count.

I remember how many women I have never met messaged me to thank me for sharing my journey with its ups and its downs.

I remember Lennox's first "love you, Mama," "you funny," and "you my queen."

I am alive, I am healthy, my loved ones are by my side and I am ready to make 2019 another year to **REMEMBER**! Who's with me? #Happy2019

"I just love how you look at life. Wishing you all the best for this new year."

Choosing how to look at life has always come naturally to me. This was particularly true after I moved to the U.S. I had no money, no friends and no family. My life started from zero and no day was an easy one. It was then that I learned that there were many reasons to give thanks each day. First, I was healthy. That, in itself, was an amazing blessing. Second, while I had nothing, I was in the land of opportunity. Every single day I had the chance to go out in the world and build a beautiful life. The fact that that was even an option blew my mind with gratefulness daily.

Fast forward to the end of 2018. The year was marked by much more than those two miscarriages. Of course, there were lots of lows that came from those two pivotal events. But there were also lots of highs in my life that year. Lennox was healthy and becoming his own little person. Never had I been more in love with him.

My husband and I had grown tremendously strong after going through so much in such a short period of time. We had learned to put pride aside, communicate better and overall become better partners and teammates. Above all, we had learned to love each other better. This path of ours had shown us that it is easy to adore your partner when things are good and beautiful. But there is a special kind of love that is born after going through darkness together. My husband had seen me at my worst, yet he kept choosing me every single day. Not only that, but he kept helping me pick up my broken pieces and rebuild myself. And each time, I came out of it a stronger person.

While that had been my 2018, I must confess that the comment about having 'a year to forget' hurt me. It made me realize that there was a downside to having been so open about my struggles. Some people had begun to see me only for my pain. The heartache I was going through had become my identity for some.

This was a painful realization, because it happened exactly when I was starting to feel as if I could forgive myself and stop thinking about my body as defective. To learn that people may only be seeing me for the pain came as a very unpleasant surprise.

Luckily, I received that comment while on vacation in Spain, surrounded by the people I love the most. For the first time in 16 years, I was going to spend New Year's Eve with my mom and brothers. Not only that, we were going to celebrate my mom's 70th birthday only a few days after that. The trip was exactly what my soul needed. Being home with the people who know me the best was incredibly healing. Watching Lennox bond with my family, having dinner together, walking the streets in the evenings… I felt nothing but peace and comfort.

The unfortunate comment was quickly forgotten, as I allowed myself to simply be in the moment and stop being 'Sandy the Warrior,' 'Sandy the Miscarriage Awareness Girl,' or anyone else. I was just me and I needed that. As much as I needed to share my journey and hopefully empower other families, I also needed to simply be me at times.

If you decide to share your miscarriage experience, you may find yourself in a similar position as I did. It is scary to think that people may label you. And that sometimes they might label you as a woman who is failing at something that should happen naturally. It is painful enough to feel that way about yourself, let alone have others thinking that way.

But one of the biggest lessons I have learned after four years and four miscarriages is that the good you do by sharing your story far outweighs any unfortunate label a few people may give you. With that being said, if you choose to share, do it on your own terms and in your own time. Only you know when you are ready to do so. You cannot and should not try to save the world with broken wings. Allow your pain and your healing to take place before even considering how you can help others with their own healing.

It is my hope that many of you reading this will find healing within these pages. But that is not my only hope. The world needs to learn the lessons about loss, and I am but one voice. So it is my hope that you might also find the strength to share your journey with others. And by sharing your story, you also find peace in the process.

Who knows how my story would have gone if I had stayed silent. God knows I am glad that I did not choose that path.

CYNTHIA'S STORY

The posts you have shared talking about your miscarriages have always brought me to tears. I had a silent miscarriage a few months ago. I am now 12 weeks pregnant. Today, I have my nuchal translucency scan and I am really nervous. The last time I went to have this test done, it revealed that my baby girl no longer had a heartbeat. Your posts are so inspiring and helpful. Please do not stop sharing them. Women like me need women like you.

Join the movement. Share these stories so that we all have a voice. #TheLightAfterLoss

☉   @siramara
f   Sandy Bodeau
🐦   @sanbodeau

CHAPTER 28

CARRIE UNDERWOOD SENT ME A SIGN

February 11, 2019

Do you believe in signs? I do! I think that life is always reminding us to never give up. Sometimes, we just miss it if we put our focus in the wrong place.

A few weeks back, I told my husband I was done trying to have another baby. I felt drained. Drained from the heartbreak of three losses in less than two years. Drained from working so hard in staying faithful but getting my hopes down month after month. My hope tank was really getting to an empty point.

Then, a few days back, I randomly found an interview where @carrieunderwood confessed she had had three miscarriages after the birth of her first son. And I saw this interview only two days after she welcomed her second baby!! There was MY sign.

There will be times when you want something SO badly that your heart will hurt at the possibility of not getting it. And there will also be times when you'll feel like you can't be hopeful anymore. Then, it's time to open your eyes really big and find YOUR sign.

> *"I am anxiously waiting for the day when I open my Instagram app and see your pregnancy announcement. Your loyal followers know how hard you are fighting to make your dream happen. God's timing is perfect and he gives his toughest battles to his strongest warriors. Do not punish yourself and never lose hope. We are all with you,"*

There we were, six months after my fourth miscarriage. I was not the only one feeling drained. He never told me, but I could see the pressure in my husband's eyes. Month after month, our intimacy was becoming more and more mechanical. The deep desire of having another child was slowly killing our desire for each other. I am embarrassed to admit that I had been looking at him for months as the man who was going to get me pregnant and not my lover. We were crazy in love and our trials to conceive were making us forget that.

As soon as this became obvious, I decided that I was done trying to have another baby. Our relationship was too important to me. We had grown so much as a couple. I was not about to have the one thing that brought us closer together be the thing to cause distance between us. I wanted our relationship back. We had lost too much during the last three years. I did not want to lose my bond with my husband.

Days before that post, I had booked a trip to the Florida Keys to celebrate Lennox's second birthday. Well, we were actually celebrating all of our birthdays, since the three of us have birthdays in the same week. The trip was my attempt to escape reality and remember how we were before all the pain we had been going through. And it worked. We spent our days walking around the hotel's marina, eating way more delicious food than we needed, and lounging at the pool. It really was a fantastic way to celebrate life and to reconnect as a couple.

My husband's actual birthday was two days after our Keys trip, and I took him out to a wonderful new place where the manager hosted us. We had one of the best meals we had had in a very long time. The hotel was actually hosting us for the weekend and we had a wonderful night at the hotel's rooftop. It had been literally months since we had gone out to have drinks together. That night felt like we were back to our dating days. In between all our sadness and efforts to reach our dream to grow our family, we had found each other again.

On that high, I decided to also celebrate my sweet love on Valentine's day, a week after his birthday. We went back to the same restaurant/rooftop. It just felt right. We had found our groove as a couple back there, and we wanted the momentum to keep going. We always say that we do not like celebrating Valentine's Day – because we truly celebrate our life daily – but this year felt special to me. After so much heartbreak, I was ready to look at life in a much simpler way. So, yes, that year, I wanted to be corny and celebrate our love on that particular day.

What I did not know was that just a few weeks later, I would be celebrating something else: a pregnancy! It was on that Valentine's Day and three days after my post about the Carrie Underwood 'sign' that I became pregnant with our daughter. It had happened! After months of tension, sadness, and uncertainty, my body gave me what I had been wanting for the past months and it did it when I stopped putting pressure on it to do so.

As I had said to my girlfriends so many times before: "Pregnancy is the most natural process there is. You cannot force it. Do not stress about it and allow your body to do it." Now, I knew that there were many women who struggled with getting pregnant. But I also knew that I was not one of them, meaning my recent issues were probably due to the stress of trying to force the issue. For the past few months, I had forgotten that very advice I had given many times before. The minute I allowed Mother Nature to take over, without obsessing about it, it happened! We were going to have the baby we had been dreaming of for over a year!

TANIA'S STORY

I am really sorry to bother you with my sadness but I cannot help but thinking about you after what just happened to me. I was expecting my second child. I was 10 weeks pregnant. Yesterday, I started bleeding out of nowhere. I literally felt as if my body was trying to get rid of my baby while I tried to do all I could to prevent it. I lost my baby.

I do not know why this had to happen. I do not understand. I took good care of myself. I ate healthy. I got plenty of rest. I already loved that baby and he/she was stolen from me. I am really sad and really angry. I am afraid of how angry I am feeling.

My little boy is one and a half and I do not want him to see me this way, but I cannot help but feeling like I am about to go into the darkest of places. The pain is so real even though I never got to meet this baby. Please, tell me if I will ever heal from this pain. Right now, it does not feel like I ever will.

Join the movement. Share these stories so that we all have a voice. #TheLightAfterLoss

@siramara
Sandy Bodeau
@sanbodeau

CHAPTER 29

FINDING NEW LIGHT

May 12, 2019

#WaitingForYouBabyGirl "If your path is more difficult it's because your calling is higher."

To all the mamas, you are WARRIORS and I'm honored to be one of you. Happy Mother's Day.

> *"Congratulations!!!! I am so very happy for you!!! You are so blessed after waiting so long and after enduring your losses!! Sending much love to you and your beautiful family!!! Can't wait to see her!!"*

And so it was that I announced that we were expecting another baby. It was Mother's Day, and I was 12 weeks pregnant. The joyful picture announcing the pregnancy hid the fact that I had spent the last few weeks worried sick about having yet another miscarriage. And that was not the only secret it hid.

My worry and concern about this pregnancy began from the start. So much so, that my doctor had decided to see me weekly just to give me peace of mind. We had simply had too much heartbreak and too many failures.

During my week 11 appointment, my doctor told me that I was almost out of the danger zone and asked me if I was finally feeling better about this pregnancy. She said to me: "I have zero concerns about this pregnancy. When will you start feeling better about it?" I broke down crying and confessed that I would not feel better until I had that baby in my arms. The last couple of years had stolen my ability to be excited about a pregnancy. They had stolen my ability to believe that I could carry another pregnancy to term. All I had left was my faith that it could happen, but that faith was nearly consumed by fear.

In spite of all the nerves and doubts, I had developed an amazing bond with my doctor. Seeing her so confident about this pregnancy suddenly made me stop being fearful. I went home that day feeling like another person. My baby was going to be okay.

Three days after that appointment, we were supposed to receive the results from the genetic screening. This was a test that had become popular as a way to learn the sex of your baby earlier than via ultrasound. But, after all my losses, this was a test that I needed to 'pass' to have true peace of mind.

My husband called me, sounding excited. "I have the doctor on the line, she wants to talk to us." He did not realize what was immediately clear to me. She did not want to talk to us 'just' because she had the results. I started hyperventilating and told my husband: "That is not good news."

Minutes later, my amazing doctor was on the phone to deliver shocking news to us once again. Our baby had a nine out of ten chance of having Down syndrome. My heart stopped. I could not speak or think. We agreed to go see the specialist right away and hung up.

Silently, I walked towards our bedroom while Lennox napped in his. Closing the door behind me, I threw the phone against my bed and fell on my knees crying. A pillow muffled my screams so that Lennox could not hear me sobbing. It was as if my heart was breaking into a thousand pieces. I cried inconsolably.

The peace that I had finally found within this pregnancy was shattered. Three days was all it lasted. For three precious days, I had been able to enjoy what I thought would be an uneventful pregnancy once and for all. And now that peace was gone.

An hour after the call, my husband, Lennox and I headed to the specialist. In such a haze, it had not occurred to me to make arrangements for someone to watch Lennox. Walking into the specialist's office, I told myself, "Someone is that one out of ten."

A technician did an ultrasound and the doctor came minutes after. "I wish I had better news." The air was taken from my lungs as I began sobbing again. This time much more calmly as I did not want Lennox to see me. "The physical traits I see are consistent with Down syndrome."

Anger raged and boiled within my body. I was angry that, after all my miscarriages, I was now getting my heart broken again. Angry that it was this doctor, and not my beloved obstetrician, who was delivering this devastating news. Angry that my heart was being shattered in a room full of strangers. This had to be a nightmare. It was not possible that this was actually happening.

The doctor explained to me that I could take an invasive test to confirm what was suspected. The chorionic villus sampling (CVS) is a prenatal test used to detect birth defects, genetic diseases, and other problems during pregnancy. During the test, a small sample of cells is taken from the placenta where it attaches to the wall of the uterus. I agreed to take the test right then and there, because I needed a definite answer.

As best as I could, I held it together as the doctor introduced a needle through my belly to collect the cells. My little boy watched cartoons a few feet away, unaware of what was happening. I wanted to scream. I wanted to cry. I wanted to run away from that room and pretend that I had never been there. I wanted to unhear all of the words that we had just heard. Instead, I was numb and frozen on the table as the test was performed.

The results would take a week. And the fear of the unknown took me to the darkest place I have ever been. Four nights in a row I cried myself to sleep. But on the fifth day post-diagnosis, I woke up, enlightened. There is no other way to describe it. As my eyes opened that morning, I stared at the ceiling and thought: "Have you forgotten that you are still pregnant? If you are feeling this sadness so intensely, so is your baby. This stops today." I will forever be grateful for that moment. It was then that I started my own personal transformation to becoming the mom that I need to be for this baby. Our baby whose Down syndrome diagnosis was confirmed a few days later.

The last few days had been so shocking that we had not even asked about the sex of our baby. In spite of everyone assuming that our baby was a boy (based on the rapid heart rate), my gut told me that I was expecting a little girl. So did my husband's. When texting my doctor with an update on how I was feeling post diagnosis, I ended by asking: "Do you happen to remember the sex of our baby?" "I do, Sandy. It is a girl."

On that day, I decided to give our daughter a name that for two decades I had wanted to honor. It was the name of my Abuela. That was also the day I let go of the baby that I thought I was having. Instead, I embraced the baby we were having: Mara. It was time to use the strength given to me by so many others who found comfort in how I shared my journey.

When a woman wrote to tell me that I had given her hope to keep trying to have a baby, I found light in darkness. When a woman confessed that she had never spoken about her miscarriage, but after seeing my posts was compelled to do so, I found light in darkness. When a woman messaged me right after losing a baby to tell me that she knew she was going to be okay because she had been following my journey, I found light in darkness.

ISABELLA'S STORY

My miscarriage happened on January 15, 1977. I was about 13 weeks pregnant. I have never forgotten that day. I still think 'what if' and the 'why'. Particularly as July 15 approaches; my estimated due date.

I now find myself having to help a dear niece that has gone through a loss herself. She was also 13 weeks pregnant. Even though I know all about the pain, the questions, the deep hole that miscarriage leaves in your heart, the silence and isolation, the pretending to be OK because life goes on, I am happy to have found you on Instagram to be able to show her another woman that she may relate to during this hard time.

———————

Join the movement. Share these stories so that we all have a voice. #TheLightAfterLoss

@siramara
Sandy Bodeau
@sanbodeau

CHAPTER 30

REDEFINING LIGHT

October 23, 2019

There is a Spanish saying that says: "There is only one mother." But that was never my case. I was so very lucky to get two: my actual mom and my grandma. The two most important women in my life.

My grandma was an angel on Earth and my mother is the epitome of the word warrior. And that's what I hope my little girl will become: a kind angel capable of standing up for herself and pushing through adversity. A mix of the two.

After the toughest two years of my life, it is with tears in my eyes that I introduce you to my daughter, named after my grandma and my mama. Ladies and gentlemen, born on 10/22/19, 9.5 lbs, 20.5": it is my honor to introduce you all to my daughter Mara Victoria aka #Wondergirl.

> *"Beautiful!!! We are going to share the same birthday ... I predict that you will be an angel and a warrior, but in addition to that, you will be brave and a protagonist, because that is how we are born on this day."*

My experience with multiple miscarriages, and opening up about them, had become among the most meaningful experiences of my life. They laid the groundwork for me to take this recent news and search for the meaning and the lessons within. The last three years had shown me that light does not only appear at the end of the tunnel. There are places within the darkness that provide great opportunities for growth. It was because of these experiences that I knew, beyond the initial darkness that I endured when we received Mara's diagnosis, this new development would lead to the brightest light that ever was.

That was the lesson I learned at three months pregnant, having just received the diagnosis. And now that my little girl has been born, it has been confirmed. My pregnancy with Mara was a transformational process for me. The six months of pregnancy following the diagnosis literally turned me into a different person. And I would like to think I am a better person.

We were incredibly blessed along the way. Appointment after appointment, with an amazing team of specialists, we continued to receive encouraging news. Mara defied the odds by not having heart, digestive or other serious physical issues. And learning of any other potential limitations were only viewed as a challenge. That simply became the fuel for my desire to give both my children my very best and as many opportunities in life as I could get for them.

Mara's diagnosis taught me so much about life and about love. It taught me that very few things are truly important, and those are the ones that really matter. It also revealed how little I cared about conventional ideas about what is 'normal' and what is not. And it reminded me how our individuality is what makes us all special. It is not going to be any different for our little girl. Above it all, I knew that Mara was going to be born into a great family. That she would be happy. That she would be endlessly loved. And that her life would be a life worth living, and celebrating.

Every single day, I learn from the women who open their hearts to me on social media. They feed my light. It is my hope that my story can do the same for you. Someone once told me that "as much as hurt people hurt people, healed people heal people." And that is exactly what I decided to do with my recurrent pregnancy loss experience.

My healing came from learning that I could make an impact on others by sharing how difficult my motherhood journey has been. The end of my journey does not look like I thought it would look. And, yet, I could have never anticipated how much more meaningful, impactful, and overall amazing it turned out to be.

Hundreds of times I had asked myself, "Why is this my journey? What do I need to learn from it?" Finally, I have the answer. I had to go through that journey to become my most vulnerable self. It was through that vulnerability that I learned that serving others is what gives your life true meaning. And, ultimately, because I had found purpose in helping others previously, I now know that by sharing Mara's journey it will help other families finding themselves in our current position.

This peaceful perspective I have is owed in large part to Luz María, Noelia, Paula, Elisabeth, Ruth, Penelope, Beatrice, Daniela, Julene, Vanessa, Shannon, Nadia, Jennifer, Carrie, Adriana, Diana, Elle, Barbara, Catherine, Juliana, Kim, Susan, Christina, Nora, Tamara, Camila, Ana Maria, Cynthia, Tania, Isabella, Kristen and the hundreds of others who have shared with me their journey of pregnancy loss. They taught me about finding light after loss. I cried reading each and every one of the messages that I received through the years. In fact, I still do. They have helped me grow as a person and learn that we can use our pain and turn it into healing for someone else. That purpose can be found during the worst of times. That 'light' means many different things depending on how we choose to look at our experiences.

On that note, here is the last story that I want to share. My niece Kristen has not experienced pregnancy loss. But her story could not be a better example of what finding light after loss means. The loss of a life you pictured having (whether or not that includes a pregnancy) deserves a mourning process, and this book was written to help the world understand that. Above it all, this book was written to help others find light in the most unexpected places. Just like we have with our pregnancy loss journey and later with Mara's diagnosis, Kristen beautifully shows how life's unplanned turns can also bring the most beautiful light after loss.

KRISTEN'S STORY

As I look at that couple in our wedding pictures, I am filled with emotion. They were so full of hope and excitement about their future. So grateful and joyful about the gift they had just been given…a beautiful marriage! And so blissfully unaware of any possibility of heartache or longing. I hardly recognize them.

Sadly, the exciting plan we had to be parents on that day almost 10 years ago has yet to come to fruition. Our arms ache to hold a sweet child of our own, but my body has not yet been able to do what it was created to do… to bear life. The grief of not having our deepest desires met is enormous.

The waiting has been tortuous: the ups and downs every month – the grueling roller coaster of hope and disappointment, the struggle with wanting to grasp and control to 'make this happen' in our timing, and hearing others' opinions about what we should do because time is running short, and most of all, carrying the deep ache of desire, and the sorrow that unfulfillment brings.

This has taken a toll over the years, and we have become weary and weak. Weary with how much effort it takes for us to attempt what others can seemingly achieve without even trying. And weak in hope that our dream of being parents will ever come to be.

However, we have also become stronger. Stronger in our marriage, stronger in our faith, stronger in our surrender, and stronger in our desire to be parents.

Thankfully, we are not the same couple we were 10 years ago. A wise man once expressed how waiting increases our heart's capacity to love, and this wait has done just that! Our hearts are expanding every day in love for each other; in gratitude for the many gifts we have been given, and in recognition of how important and treasured a child is… how honored we would be if we were given this most precious gift.

Our hearts and our arms are open… however that may come to be

———————

Join the movement. Share these stories so that we all have a voice. #TheLightAfterLoss

@siramara

Sandy Bodeau

@sanbodeau

ACKNOWLEDGEMENTS

Mama because I simply cannot imagine how I would have ever been able to walk this path without having you pick up my broken pieces, time and time again. I would be absolutely lost without you. My children are beyond blessed that you are their Abuela.

Manu for always believing that I can reach the stars and for being my forever best friend and soulmate.

Oscar for having been my everything and more through childhood.

Papa - I wish so bad that you could see the woman that your little girl has turned into.

Abuela - I will never stop missing you and love the fact that I will now get to see you daily in my baby girl.

Tia Pili because you always told me "I know that you will not just work 9-5 at a desk in Madrid," and I so wish that you would have gotten to see how very right you were. You knew what I was capable of way before I did. I miss you terribly.

Axier for being the most wonderful cousin my kids could have. You will forever be the first baby I madly fell in love with!

Dr. Anna T. Davis, my beloved obstetrician. You are a true gift to the medical field. There would have been no light to follow without your unconditional support throughout this journey.

Colleen McGinn because you are one of the biggest blessings that the U.S. has given me; only second to avocado!

Abel Arana because one can never have enough big brothers and you are the best one life could have given me.

José María Lucena because you will forever hold the record for the person I've loved the fastest.

Anabelle Blum for having been my TV mentor, my cheerleader and my secret keeper any time I've needed one.

Barbie Musa for making me believe more and more daily that a true friend is a treasure.

Luis Aponte for absolutely everything you are to me and my family. I love you like a love song!

Alice Yacaman for always being so close to me, no matter how long we may go without seeing each other.

Cynthia D Costa for always having me in your thoughts and prayers when I need it the most.

Aileen Abella for having one of the most generous hearts I have ever seen and always be willing to share it with me.

Lilian Santini for helping me with the amazing cover of this book but, most importantly, for helping me any time I need a friend and making me feel like we have family next door.

Zuleyka Rivera for all these years of friendship, after meeting during one of my favorite TV projects to date.

Bob Schuchts for your guidance and compassion.

Carrie Daunt for allowing me to learn from you and always having wise words of advice.

Kristen Blake for inspiring me endlessly without even trying. The end of this book is incredible thanks to you and your beautiful heart. You are a gem!

U.S. Senator Tom Carper for giving me my first big job in the United States and for teaching me that serving others is what makes our life impactful.

Amy Hudson for helping me rediscover the student that I was growing up – which led me to a wildly beautiful professional life.

Luz María Doria for not laughing at me when I told you that I wanted to write a book and actually encouraging me to do so. Having your foreword in my first book will forever be one of my biggest professional accomplishments. I am forever thankful for your willingness to mentor me.

Lennox Ryan for teaching me for the first time what unconditional love means and for showing me daily what true happiness looks like. May the world never, ever cut your beautiful wings, my precious boy!

Mara Victoria (aka Wondergirl) for changing my life forever. For opening my eyes to a better world and making me stronger, wiser and overall better as a human. We are going to change the world, baby girl!

Richard. My love. My partner. My biggest cheerleader. For our love, for our life, and for having been so incredibly vested in this project. It could never have happened without you.

To all the women who shared their pregnancy loss story with me. You gave me a voice and a purpose when you showed me how much isolation there was around this topic. I pray that your bravery encourages many others to continue this very needed conversation about miscarriage in an open and compassionate way.

And, last but not least, YOU reading this book. Whether you have experienced loss or have a loved one who has, thank you for trusting me with your heart. I have given you mine within these pages.

ABOUT THE AUTHOR

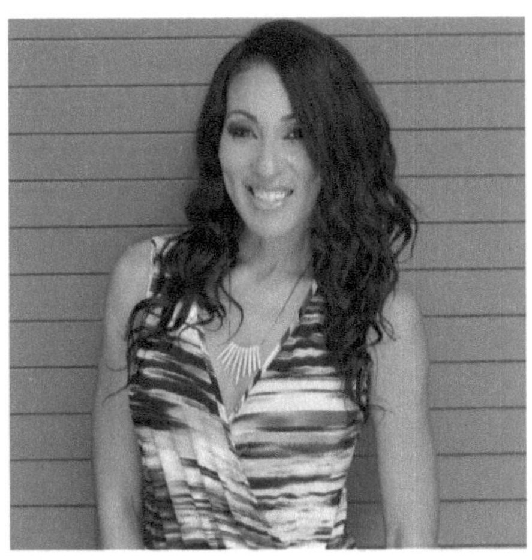

SANDY BODEAU is a Renaissance woman who is proving that the American dream is alive and well. Having arrived in the United States from her hometown of Madrid (Spain) with just $800 and no English vocabulary, Sandy went on to graduate top of her college class, not once but twice. Her optimistic, engaging, and caring personality made her an outstanding member of U.S. Senator Tom Carper's team, advocating for constituents facing challenges with federal programs. When Sandy started her own jewelry business, Sira&Mara, those same skills enabled her to quickly build a strong and loyal customer base.

It was precisely those same customers who encouraged Sandy to start a personal style blog. The success of her blog led Sandy to be discovered by a TV producer in 2014. Since then, Sandy has become a regular contributor in Spanish speaking TV shows, including Univision's Despierta América. As a blogger, Sandy has worked in multiple campaigns with some of the biggest brands in the world, such as Disney, and her work has been recognized by major publications including Vanity Fair and Cosmopolitan for Latinas.